THE EXTRA POINT SERIES:

EPONYMS & BUZZWORDS

FOR USMLE

1st Edition, 2010

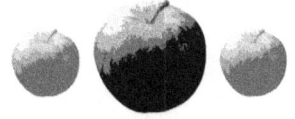

AN APPLE-A-DAY BOOKS CREATION

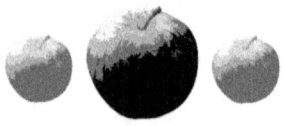

ABOUT APPLE-A-DAY BOOKS

Apple-A-Day Books was created by Ognjen "Ogi" Visnjevac and Frederick Ma as an official medical student promotion and publication company.

Realizing the incredible value of the too-often-squandered eager student mind, *Apple-A-Day Books'* goal is to create publications for three purposes: (1) to improve medical and health education; (2) to provide new and innovative public health solutions; and (3) to inspire students to do more, to advance their careers, and to take responsibility as leaders in healthcare within their own communities.

For more information about *Apple-A-Day Books*, visit:

www.AppleADayBooks.com

This book is dually dedicated:

Firstly, we dedicate this to the families, friends, peers, and loved ones of the authors, who have supported us in our many goals. We thank you from the bottom of our hearts. Your love and support has always been, and always will be sincerely appreciated.

Secondly, to all medical students everywhere – and to those interested in or have a passion for learning: the authors wrote this book for you. We congratulate each of you on your endeavor to become a health professional. Your path is not easy and requires both perseverance and diligence. Years ago, we too experienced challenges and frustrations in studying medicine. As future physicians, it is a medical students' obligation to accrue a wealth of knowledge, including that which may often confuse and frustrate us: eponyms. Time to learn is limited. It is our goal to aid fellow and future students so that they might learn medicine to a higher degree of clarity and proficiency. To you, we offer this teaching tool – this book of eponyms – and we hope that it guides you to a stronger understanding of medicine and, ultimately, to stellar USMLE scores.

EDITORS-IN-CHIEF

OGNJEN VISNJEVAC, MSIII
St. George's University, Grenada, West Indies

FREDERICK MA, MSIII
St. George's University, Grenada, West Indies

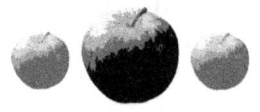

CONTENT EDITORS

NADA BOSKOVIC, MD, FACP

Visiting Professor of Immunology, University of

Northumbria, UK

STEVICA BOSKOVIC, MD, MPH

Niagara Falls, Canada

EWARLD MARSHALL, MD

Assistant Professor of Anatomy, St. George's University

School of Medicine, Grenada, West Indies

CRISTOFRE MARTIN, PhD

Professor of Biochemistry and Genetics, St. George's

University School of Medicine, Grenada, West Indies

WILLIAMS MERBS

Instructor of Anatomy, St. George's University School of

Medicine, Grenada, West Indies

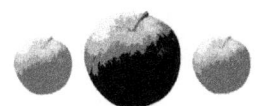

<u>ACKNOWLEDGMENTS:</u>

We would like to thank the following people for their help, ideas, inputs, and support throughout the writing and development of this book:

Dr. N. Aquino, Dr. D. Burns, Dr. F. Brahim, Dr. L. Dasso, Dr. R. Hage, M. Hanna, A. Komorowsky, T. Krunic, Dr. M. Loukas, C. Malabanan, J. McGuirk, Dr. C. Modica, Dr. C.V. Rao, D. Seidler, Family Visnjevac, & St. George's University

TABLE OF CONTENTS
& CONTRIBUTING AUTHORS

How to Get the Most Out of This Book

The purpose of *Eponyms & Buzzwords for USMLE* is to aid and ease the journey for fellow medical students. The knowledge of medicine is ever growing. With every discovery of a new disease, the contributing scientist or doctor will tag their name onto the defined syndrome or illness, thus leading to the creation of an eponym. With the long-standing history of medicine, thousands of eponyms have been created. Scientists have finished sequencing human DNA in less than a decade. With that achievement, hundreds of gene sequences have been labeled and correlated with human diseases. Lastly, doctors love giving nicknames to complex clinical signs or pathological clues as a means if simplifying communication. While such naming and classification decreases miscommunication when used properly, the similarity and sheer volume of terms may confuse and frustrate young student doctors learning medicine.

This book contains over 1900 eponyms and buzzwords. Where do we start? This book is categorized into anatomical and physiological systems. Under every system, we have subcategorized relevant eponyms into a *STAR Classification.* We have reviewed every single grueling eponym and rated their relevance and significance to USMLE examinations in numbers-of-stars. Each term can have a maximum rating of five stars and a minimum of one star. What does each star mean?

☆☆☆☆☆	5-STAR YIELD	**Must Know For Life**
☆☆☆☆	4-STAR YIELD	**Very High Yield**
☆☆☆	3-STAR YIELD	**High Yield**
☆☆	2-STAR YIELD	Technical and/or Trivial Terms, or Alternate Names for Eponymous Terminology
☆	1-STAR YIELD	

Use your stars!

Added to many eponyms, there is also a, "Don't Confuse This With," statement. There are many eponyms in medicine that may almost have the same spelling and have entirely different meanings, or similar meanings with totally different eponymous names. Take advantage of this section to solidify your knowledge and score higher on your exams. This book also contains a list of the genes you need to know for USMLE in an exclusive chapter. Do not neglect this chapter.

Lastly, if you are searching for a specific eponym, you can use our index to find your word with ease. The purpose of *Eponyms & Buzzwords for USMLE* is to ease and enhance your medical studies. *Eponyms & Buzzwords for USMLE* cannot be used as a primary learning source but a supplemental tool to make learning more enjoyable. We wish you luck and we hope this book enhances your medical education.

CHAPTER 1: ABDOMEN & GASTROINTESTINAL TRACT

Courvoisier sign (Clinical Medicine) - Head of pancreas cancer causes enlarged gallbladder. Don't Confuse This With: Cholecystitis

Charcot Triad (Clinical Medicine) – Triad of fever, jaundice, and right-upper quadrant abdominal pain suggestive of ascending cholangitis.

Crohn Disease (Pathology) - Subacute and chronic systemic inflammatory disease characterized by fibrosis, ulcers, fistulas, and noncaseating tuberculoid granulomas in the gastrointestinal tract, particularly the ileum. Don't Confuse This With: Behçet Disease/Syndrome

Giardia (Microbiology) - Parasites belonging to flagellates genus infecting the small intestines; transmissible through oral-fecal contact. Patients present with foul smelling stools.

Hirschsprung Disease (Pathology) - Congenital megacolon caused by an absence or reduced number of ENS ganglion cells in the submucosal or myenteric plexuses of the large bowel. Megacolon characterized by bowel obstruction and colonic distension.

Krukenberg Tumor (Pathology) - Gastric carcinoma that metastasizes to the ovaries. These tumor cells produce excess mucin giving it a signet-ring shape.

Meckel diverticulum (Pathology) - Congenital anomaly of the GI tract due to the persistence of the yolk stalk, which may cause bleeding intussusception, or obstruction close to the terminal ileum; may contain ectopic gastric or pancreatic mucosa. Don't Confuse This With: Meckel Cave, Cell, Disc

Peutz-Jeghers Syndrome (Pathology) - Uncommon autosomal dominant disease characterized by hamartomatous polyps of the intestinal tract, particularly the jejunum. A brown to blackish blue pigment discoloration is also present in the lips, oral mucosa, and fingers. GI malignancies are uncommonly associated, but patients often develop extra-gastrointestinal malignancies.

Ranson Criteria (Pathology) - Standard set of symptoms used to diagnose the severity of acute pancreatitis. Initial presentation includes age > 55; WBC>16,000; glucose>200; AST>250; LDH>350. Within the first 48 hours, BUN deficit increases from > 4 to >5, fluid sequestration>6 Liters, and Ca < 8mg/dL.

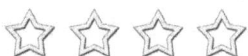

Auerbach Myenteric Plexus (Anatomy) - Enteric nervous system plexus of unmyelinated nerves and postganglionic autonomic nerve cell bodies, located between the longitudinal and circular smooth muscle layers of the esophagus, stomach and intestines. Auerbach Plexus communicates with the submucosal plexus to coordinate muscle and chyme motility in the gastrointestinal tract. Don't Confuse This With: Meissner Plexus

Barrett Esophagus (Pathology) - Chronic peptic ulceration of lower esophagus with tissue metaplasia caused by long term esophagitis, gastroesophageal reflux disease, and adenocarcinoma. Don't Confuse This With: Eagle-Barrett Syndrome

Boa Sign (Clinical Medicine) - Pain in the right subscapular region indicating cholecystitis.

Boerhaave Syndrome (Pathology) - Grave form of Mallory-Weiss Syndrome, which is characterized by a rupture of the lower esophagus causing gastric contents to empty into the mediastinum. It is commonly seen in eating disorders like bulimia.

Cullen Sign (Clinical Medicine) - Circumferential ecchymoses of the umbilicus characteristic of major intraperitoneal hemorrhaging (due to ruptured ectopic pregnancy or hemorrhaging pancreatitis). Don't Confuse This With: Blumberg Sign

Cushing Ulcer (Pathology) - Esophageal, gastric, or duodenal acute ulcer often resulting in gastrointestinal bleeding; caused by increased intracranial pressure due to neurosurgery or head trauma. Don't Confuse This With: Cushing Disease, Reaction, Syndrome, Triad; Curling Ulcer

Ulcer Flexner Disease (Pathology) - Infection caused by Shigella, characterized by intestinal inflammation and pain, diarrhea with blood and mucus. Transmission is usually from fecal contamination of food and water.

Grey Turner sign (Clinical Medicine) - Abdominal areas of discoloration indicative of acute hemorrhagic pancreatitis or other retroperitoneal hemorrhages

Kantor string sign (Clinical Medicine) - Radiographic finding: narrowing of the lumen is seen as a thin Barium line ending at the ileocecal junction. Commonly seen in regional Crohn's Disease.

Lembert Suture (Clinical Medicine) - The second row of the Czerny-Lembert intestinal suture, including collagenous submucosal layer of intestine but not penetrating the lumen.

Mallory-Weiss Syndrome (Pathology) - Laceration of the gastroesophageal mucosa causing potentially lethal hemorrhaging; often presents in patients with chronic alcoholism and induced by rigorous vomiting.

McBurney Point/Sign (Clinical Medicine) - Point on the right side situated one third of the distance from the anterior superior iliac spine to the umbilicus. Tenderness is indicative of appendicitis or ectopic pregnancy.

Meissner Plexus (Histology) - Enteric nervous system plexus of unmyelinated nerves that is present in the submucosa of the intestinal tract. Don't Confuse This With: Auerbach Plexus, Myenteric Plexus

Murphy Sign (Clinical Medicine) - for acute cholecystitis where inserting the fingertips just below the right costal margin in the mid-clavicular line while the patient takes a deep breath will elicit tenderness and the patient will immediately stop inspiration

Obturator Sign (Clinical Medicine) - Test for acute appendicitis in which the patient experiences pain in the right-sided iliac fossa while moving the right leg towards the right shoulder against resistance.

Schatzki Ring (Anatomy) - Inferior esophageal rings and webs which are often responsible for periodic food obstruction.

Reynold Pentad (Pathology) - Combination of five symptoms seen in cholangitis: jaundice, fever, and abdominal pain in the right superior quadrant (Charcot Triad) with hypotension and altered mental status. Don't Confuse This With: Reynolds Syndrome

Yellow Fever (Microbiology) - Tropical viral hepatitis caused by Flavivirus carried by mosquitoes with symptoms including jaundice, high fever, and black vomit.

Zenker Diverticulum (Pathology) - Esophageal mucosa membrane out pouching between the inferior pharyngeal constrictor and the cricopharyngeus muscle. Associated symptoms may include dysphagia and esophageal obstruction; also see Killian triangle. Don't Confuse This With: Zenker Degeneration

Barrett Epithelium (Histology) - Columnar esophageal cells present in Barrett esophagus; metaplastic response causing stratified cuboidal cells of lower esophagus to change due to gastroesophageal reflux.

Bernstein test (Clinical Medicine) - A test commonly performed in the diagnosis of GERD. It is an acid perfusion test of the esophagus using HCL, which will produce chest pain in patients with heartburn.

Bouveret syndrome (Pathology) - gallstone impaction within the duodenum causing a gastric outlet obstruction.

Castle Intrinsic Factor (Physiology) - Essential binding factor produced by gastric parietal cells for B12 absorption in the ileum.

Chagas Disease (Pathology) - Parasitic disease caused by protozoa *Trypanosoma cruzi* and which has been inoculated into the host by the Reduviid bug (defecates near bite) in South and Central America. Acute presentation includes dermatitis of affected region (Romana sign if near eye), fever, and swollen lymph nodes. Cardiomyopathy, megacolon and megaesophagus are common chronic presentations. Gastrointestinal tract megaviscera is due to myenteric plexus damage from *T. cruzi*.

Curling Ulcer (Pathology) - Acute gastric or duodenal ulcer subsequent to severe skin burns. Can be accompanied by rectal bleeding commencing 4-10 days following the burn. Don't Confuse This With: Cushing Ulcer

Dance Sign (Clinical Medicine) - Sign of intestinal retraction in the region of the right iliac fossa due to ileocecal intussusception. Don't Confuse This With: Dunphy Sign

Dieulafoy Lesion (Pathology) – A tortuous arteriole located in the submucosa of the stomach or duodenum (1st and 2nd parts) that erodes and results in an uncommon cause of acute upper gastrointestinal bleeding.

FAP (Pathology) - Familial Adenomatous Polyposis: Autosomal dominant condition characterized by hundreds of colonic polyps with about a 100% probability of developing malignant colorectal cancer. Mutation of APC gene on 5q is responsible for this disorder. Don't Confuse This With: FGID

Fruity odor (Clinical Medicine) - Ketone bodies circulating in blood during prolonged starvation and diabetic ketoacidosis (DM1)

GERD (Pathology) - Gastroesophageal Reflux Disorder: Reduced function of the Lower Esophageal Sphincter causing chronic backflow of gastric acid into the esophagus. GERD can lead to esophagitis, ulcers, esophageal stricture, and Barrett esophagus.

Ivor Lewis esophogectomy (Clinical Medicine) - Two-stage procedure in which first part involves using part of the patient's stomach to form a new esophagus. The second stage involves removing the diseased esophagus and replacing it with the newly formed one.

J tube (Clinical Medicine) - A feeding tube inserted through jejunostomy.

Kiener disease (Pathology) - chronic persistent hepatitis due to bile duct obstruction via large peripheral lymphoid follicles.

Killian Triangle (Anatomy) - A triangular area of weakness between the inferior pharyngeal constrictor and the UES (cricopharyngeus muscle) due to a normal sparseness of muscle fibers. It can be a site of Zenker diverticulum.

König disease (Pathology) - Is a GI syndrome characterized by a distended abdomen, constipation or diarrhea, and episodes of colic.

Laugier Hernia (Pathology) - A hernia through an opening in the lacunar (Gimberlat) ligament

Lynch I Syndrome (Pathology) - An autosomal dominant trait causing a familial tendency for colorectal cancer. Right-sided colorectal cancer is more common and has an early onset. Don't Confuse This With: Lynch-Wiersma Syndrome, Lynch II Syndrome

Lynch II Syndrome (Pathology) - An autosomal dominant trait causing a familial tendency for both colorectal cancer and extra intestinal cancer, predominantly of the female reproductive tract. Don't Confuse This With: Lynch-Wiersma Syndrome, Lynch I Syndrome

Mallory-Weiss Lesion (Pathology) - Esophageal mucosal laceration seen in Mallory-Weiss Syndrome. Don't Confuse This With: Mallory Bodies

Morrison pouch (Anatomy) - Hepatorenal recess, which separates the liver and right kidney; potential space that may fill due to hemoperitoneum.

Nissen fundoplication (Clinical Medicine) - Surgical treatment for gastroesophageal reflux disease. Involves using a part of the gastric muscle to produce a new sphincter at the lower end of the esophagus.

Norwalk Virus (Pathology) - Type of calcivirus that is largely responsible for non-bacterial gastroenteritis.

Peyer Patches (Histology) - Group of lymph follicles present in the lamina propria of the ileum beneath the M cells.

Plummer Vinson Syndrome (Pathology) - Condition characterized by microcytic hypochromic anemia accompanied by deterioration of the oral, glossopharyngeal, and esophageal mucous membranes. Dysphagia is also present due to the development of esophageal webs. Don't Confuse This With: Plummer Adenoma, Disease, Sign

Rigler Sign (Clinical Medicine) - Also called "double wall sign" because gas is present on both sides of the intestinal wall in an abdominal x-ray; characteristic of pneumoperitoneum. Don't Confuse This With: Rigler Triad

Rigler Triad (Pathology) - Triad of symptoms associated with gallstone ileus. Patient presents with an enlarged small intestine, gas in the biliary system, and calcified ectopic gallstones. Don't Confuse This With: Rigler Sign

Rovsing Sign (Clinical Medicine) - Sign indicative of appendicitis: pain in the right lower quadrant upon left side palpation. Right-sided rebound tenderness also present.

Scarpa Fascia (Anatomy) - The deep elastic layer of the superficial abdominal fascia. Don't Confuse This With: Scarpa's Fluid, Foramina, Ganglion, Membrane, Sheath, Staphyloma, Triangle

Schilling Test (Clinical Medicine) - Two stage test using radioactive cobalamin (B12) to distinguish between pernicious anemia and intestinal malabsorption.

Treitz, Ligament of (Anatomy) - Smooth muscle that attaches the duodeno-jejunal flexure to the diaphragm and is an important landmark to identify when looking for malrotation of the gastrointestinal tract. This anatomical structure separates upper-GI from lower-GI bleeds. Don't Confuse This With: Treitz Fascia

Valentino Sign (Clinical Medicine) – Pain and guarding in the right lower quadrant of the abdomen, due to retroperitoneal perforation of a duodenal ulcer. Don't Confuse This With: Appendicitis

Vater, Ampulla of (Anatomy) - Canal shared by the common bile and pancreatic ducts. Don't Confuse This With: Papilla of Vater

Warthin Tumor (Pathology) - Uncommon, benign parotid gland tumor known as papillary cystadenoma lymphomatosum. Patient presents with a mass at the angle of the jaw. Don't Confuse This With: Sjogren Syndrome, Mumps

Waxy cast (Pathology) - Substance found in the urine in patients with renal disease.

Whipple Disease (Pathology) - This a rare disease caused by Tropheryma whipplei. It causes malabsorption in the gastrointestinal tract but can become a systemic infection as well. Diseased tissue is filled with "foam cells".

Whipple Procedure (Clinical Medicine) - A pancreatoduodenectomy with cholecystectomy and partial bile duct excision.

Whitehead Operation (Clinical Medicine) - Surgery involving excising hemorrhoids using incisions above and below associated veins, thus normal mucosa could be pulled downwards and sutured to skin.

Allingham ulcer (Pathology) - Another name for an anal fissure. Don't Confuse This With: hemorrhoids

Amussat operation (Clinical Medicine) - Surgical procedure for creation of an orifice for a colostomy bag in the lumbar region in the case of an obstructed or absent colon.

Amyand hernia (Pathology) - Rare form of inguinal hernia (less than 1%) where the appendix is incarcerated and ruptured in the hernial sac, eliciting symptoms of appendicitis. Don't Confuse This With: Other hernias

Babington Disease (Pathology) - See Osler-Rendu-Weber Syndrome.

Balance Sign (Clinical Medicine) - A tender mass that is usually present in the left upper quadrant due to spleen hematoma.

Bant Syndrome (Pathology) - A condition in which noncirrhotic splenomegaly, hypersplenism and portal hypertension arise after a subclinical occlusion of the portal vein. The syndrome usually only develops years after the occlusive event.

Cajal, Interstitial Cells of (ICC's) (Histology) - Fibroblast-like ENS pacemaker cells located between the longitudinal and circular smooth muscle layers of the intestines. ICC's are responsible for coordination of gut contractions. Don't Confuse This With: Horizontal Cells of Cajal

Collis-Belsey fundoplication (Pathology) - Lengthening of esophagus

Cooper hernia (Pathology) - Femoral hernia with two sacs, one in the femoral canal and one appearing below just the skin. Don't Confuse This With: Cooper testis, cooper ligament

Dunphy Sign (Clinical Medicine) - Painful sensation during coughing; indicative of appendicitis. Don't Confuse This With: Dance Sign

Farber test (Clinical Medicine) - Use of X-ray to determine the presence of atresia in newborns gastrointestinal tract. Don't Confuse This With: Farber Disease

FGID (Pathology) - Functional Gastrointestinal Disorders: GI conditions of unknown pathology, which affect GI motor and sensory composition causing a multitude of symptoms. Example: IBS. Don't Confuse This With: FAP

Fitz syndrome (Pathology) - Acute pancreatitis episode marked by gangrenous inflammation of the pancreas, accompanied by fatty necrosis. Occurs in all ages and more common in females. Don't Confuse This With: Fitz-Hugh Curtis syndrome

Fournier gangrene (Microbiology) - Gangrene that forms on the skin surrounding the genital area (scrotum, perineum) following an operation or due to trauma. It is mostly seen in men due to the lack of drainage in the perineal region and is considered a urological emergency. It can be caused by a number of organisms (i.e. Bacteroides fragilis, E. coli, Candida species, Staphylococcus). Don't Confuse This With: Fournier Tibia, Fournier Sign, Peyronie Disease

Goldstein's hematemesis (Pathology) - See Osler-Rendu-Weber Syndrome.

Ladd Operation (Clinical Medicine) - Surgical procedure to divide Ladd band to fix obstruction of duodenum in patients with intestinal malrotation.

Laplace Forceps (Clinical Medicine) - Forceps used for approximating intestines during surgical anastomosis.

Lieberkühn, Crypts of (Histology) - Tubular glands present in the intestinal mucous membranes, which are responsible for enzyme secretion into the lumen of the small and large intestines.

Littres Hernia (Pathology) - Intestinal hernia of a Meckel diverticulum, which can lead to volvulus. Don't Confuse This With: Glands of Littre

Menetrier disease (Pathology) - Abnormal increase in the number of mucoid or glandular gastric mucosal cells. Don't Confuse This With: Meniere Disease

Niemann splenomegaly (Pathology) - Splenomegaly as a result of Niemann-Pick disease.

Oddi, Sphincter of (Anatomy) - Smooth muscle fibers surrounding the common bile duct, which control the secretions released into the duodenum.

Osler-Rendu-Weber Syndrome (Pathology) - Autosomal dominant disorder referred to as Hereditary Hemorrhagic Telangiectasis (HHT); characterized by capillary dilation in the skin and mucous membranes of the oral, nasopharyngeal, and intestinal membranes. These vessels often rupture causing nasal and gastrointestinal bleeding. Don't Confuse This With: Osler Triad; Oddi Syndrome; Peutz-Jeghers Syndrome

Rokitansky Disease I (Pathology) - Acute liver necrosis characterized by the death of the parenchymal liver cells and liver atrophy possibly due to a viral infection or chemical toxins. Don't Confuse This With: Rokitansky-Cushing Ulcer, Rokitansky-Aschoff Sinuses

Santorini, Duct of (Anatomy) - A duct that drains a part of the head of the pancreas. AKA Accessory pancreatic duct. Don't Confuse This With: Santorini Fissures, Santorini Muscle, Santorini Vein

Schmieden Disease (Pathology) - The gastric mucosa caves into the duodenum

Schmorl Jaundice (Pathology) – Kernicterus.

Spigelian Hernia (Pathology) – AKA lateral ventral hernia: herniation through the Spigelian fascia (aponeurosis), which is between the rectus abdominis muscle and the semilunar line, with high risk of bowel strangulation. Don't Confuse This With: Sister Mary Joseph Nodule

Stenson Duct (Anatomy) - Duct which drains parotid gland secretions into the oral cavity. Duct is located across from the second maxillary molar tooth.

Vater, Papilla of (Anatomy) - Nipple shaped structure, which empties the pancreaticobiliarly tree into the second portion of the duodenum. Don't Confuse This With: Ampulla of Vater

Waldenström-Kjellberg syndrome (Pathology) - See Plummer Vinson Syndrome.

Wirsüng, Duct of (Anatomy) - Principal pancreatic duct that empties into the major duodenal papilla. Don't Confuse This With: Ampulla of Vater, Papilla of Vater

Aaron sign (Clinical Medicine) - In appendicitis, continuous, applied pressure over McBurney point will eventually result in referred pain to the epigastric or substernal region. This heart/stomach pain is called Aaron's sign. Don't Confuse This With: McBurney sign, Psoas sign

Allison-Johnston disease (Pathology) - See Barrett Esophagus. Don't Confuse This With: Addison Disease

Alvarez syndrome (Pathology) - A neurological disorder resulting in bloating of the abdomen without clinical cause. Theoretically due to abnormal abdominal muscle contraction. Don't Confuse This With: Ascites, kwashiorkor

Annandale operation (Clinical Medicine) - A surgical procedure that corrects and inguinal and femoral hernia at the same time.

Asherson syndrome (Pathology) - A syndrome caused by neuromuscular discoordination resulting in severe dysphagia. Aspiration pneumonia may ensue.

Blumberg Sign (Clinical Medicine) - Abdominal pain present when constant pressure is applied and then released. Pain associated with peritonitis. Don't Confuse This With: Cullen Sign

Brunner Glands (Physiology) - Branched, coiled, tubular submucosal glands which secrete alkaline mucous into ducts which drain into intervillar crypts of the duodenum.

Carnett Test (Clinical Medicine) - Disappearance of abdominal tenderness to palpation when the anterior abdominal muscles are contracted, indicating pain of intra-abdominal origin; its persistence suggests a source in the abdominal wall, which is also indicated when tenderness is caused by gently pinching a fold of skin and fat between the thumb and forefinger.

Charcot intermittent fever (Pathology) - Fever resulting from common bile duct obstruction. Don't Confuse This With: Charcot Triad

Chaussier sign (Clinical Medicine) - Pain in epigastium due to hemorrhage into the liver capsule.

Chilaiditi Syndrome (Pathology) - Transverse colonic or small intestinal volvulus caused by the interposition of an intestinal loop between the liver and right diaphragm.

Connell suture (Clinical Medicine) - A continuous suture used for inverting the gastric or intestinal walls in performing an anastomosis.

Cronkhite-Canada Syndrome (Pathology) - Noncancerous gastrointestinal mucosal abnormality characterized by hamartomatous polyps causing a disturbance in GI absorption. Symptoms include weight loss, electrolyte/protein imbalance, diarrhea, and GI bleeding.

Patients also present with alopecia and nail atrophy. Don't Confuse This With: Crohn Disease

Czerny suture (Clinical Medicine) - Needle enters the serosa of intestine and passes out through the submucosa or muscularis, and then enters the submucosa or muscularis of the opposite side and emerges from the serosa.

Eder-Pustow bougie (Clinical Medicine) - A metal bougie (dilator device) to treat esophageal stricture. Edwardsiella (Microbiology) - A genus of opportunistic gram-negative bacteria. It is an etiologic agent of gastroenteritis in humans.

GISTS (Pathology) - Gastrointestinal Stromal Tumors: Most nonepithelial tumors present in the stomach and intestines mainly. GISTS affect differentiation of smooth muscle tissue and autonomic nerves.

Glisson Sphincter (Anatomy) - See Oddi Sphincter.

Goldstein's heredofamilial angiomatosis (Pathology) - See Osler-Rendu-Weber Syndrome.

Hirschsprung-Galant infantilism (Pathology) - See Hirschsprung Disease

Hutchinson-Weber-Peutz Syndrome (Pathology) - See Peutz-Jeghers syndrome.

Jaccoud-Osler Disease (Pathology) - Hemorrhagic telangiectasia disease that is a type of Osler-Rendu-Weber Syndrome. Don't Confuse This With: Osler Triad

Kelly Syndrome (Pathology) - See Plummer Vinson Syndrome.

Klostermann Syndrome (Pathology) - See Peutz-Jeghers syndrome.

Lane Band (Anatomy) - Congenital band adhesions in distal area of ileum.

Meyenburg Complex (Pathology) - Clustered bile ducts found in polycystic livers. Don't Confuse This With: Meyenburg Disease

Mya Disease (Pathology) - See Hirschsprung Disease.

Oddi Syndrome (Pathology) - Spasms of the Sphincter of Oddi, which parallels the symptoms of pain and jaundice seen with a common bile duct obstruction. Don't Confuse This With: Osler Syndrome

Osler's syndrome/disease (Pathology) - See Osler-Rendu-Weber Syndrome. Don't Confuse This With: Osler Triad, Oddi Syndrome

Paneth Cells (Histology) - Enzyme and protein secreting cells located in the crypts of Lieberkühn in the small intestine.

Paterson Syndrome (Pathology) - See Plummer Vinson Syndrome.

Peutz-Touraine syndrome (Pathology) - See Peutz-Jeghers syndrome.

Richter Hernia (Pathology) - See Littre's hernia. Don't Confuse This With: Richter Syndrome

Rokitansky-Aschoff Sinuses (Pathology) - Acquired herniation of the gallbladder mucosa into the muscular wall present during inflammation. Don't Confuse This With: Rokitansky-Cushing Ulcer, Rokitansky Disease

Rokitansky-Cushing Ulcer (Pathology) - See Cushing Ulcer. Don't Confuse This With: Cushing Disease, Cushing Syndrome, Curling Ulcer, Cushing Reaction

Rosenbach-Gmelin Test (Clinical Medicine) - Laboratory testing method using nitric acid to determine if bile is present in the urine.

Ruysh Disease (Pathology) - See Hirschsprung Disease.

Saegesser Sign (Clinical Medicine) - A sign indicating a splenic rupture or intracapsular bleeding, elicited by the compression of the phrenic point located along the border of the sternocleidomastoid muscle, causing excruciating pain along the lateral border of the rectus abdominis muscle. AKA phrenic-point test.

Santos Syndrome (Pathology) - Hirschsprung disease with additional symptoms to megacolon including hearing loss, renal agenesis, polydactyl, and hypertelorsim.

Schwartz Dictum (Pathology) - Dictum "No acid, No ulcer" meaning that peptic acid is the precursor of duodenal ulcers.

Seligmann Disease (Pathology) - Penetration of the small bowel lamina propria by lymphoplasmacytoid cells, which produce truncated heavy chains. Don't Confuse This With: Spigelian Hernia

Toldt, White lines of (Anatomy) - Peritoneal folds along the lateral borders of the ascending and descending colon.

Waldeyer Sheath (Anatomy) - Space between bladder wall and the intramural part of ureter.

Watertrap stomach (Anatomy) - Highly dilated and ptotic stomach with a high pyloric outlet that is suspended by gastrohepatic ligament.

Wepfer Glands (Histology) - See Brunner's Glands.

Chapter 2: Behavioral Science

Erik Erikson Stages of Psychosocial Development
(Clinical Medicine) - Stages of life that are characterized by
a psychosocial task that must be mastered in order to
mature to the next stage, with mastery of the following
stage allowing for the acquisition of the previous stage's
ego strength.

Piaget's Stages of Cognitive Development (Clinical
Medicine) - 4 stages of cognitive development:
sensorimotor, preoperational, concrete operational, and
formal operational that describe how children acquire,
arrange, and organize their experiences into constructs in
order to make sense of the environment through
assimilation and accommodation.

Asperger disorder (Pathology) – A male-dominant autistic
spectrum disorder that is less severe, has a later onset,
and is more common than autism. There is impaired social
interaction, repetitive patterns of behavior and interests,
unusual abilities, and marked deficits in pragmatics and
intonation, but no language or cognitive development
delays. Don't Confuse This With: Autism

Kanner Syndrome (Pathology) - Classified as a form of
autism. One of the major presenting symptoms is lack of
responsiveness to other people. There is an abnormality of
language and behavioral development.

Maslow Hierarchy of Needs (Clinical Medicine) - It is a theory in psychology that states that people fulfill their needs in the following order of importance: physiological, safety, love/belonging, esteem, and actualization.

Munchausen syndrome (Factitious Syndrome) (Pathology) - Artificial and self-induced lesions inflicted by self; the patient claims no responsibility for the act; a psychological condition that requires, in most cases, management with a psychiatrist. Don't Confuse This With: Munchausen syndrome by proxy

Munchausen's syndrome by proxy (Pathology) - AKA Factitious Disorder: A psychiatric condition in which a caregiver repeatedly simulates an illness in a child for medical attention; a type of child abuse. Don't Confuse This With: Munchausen syndrome, Malingering

Kohlberg's Stages of Moral Reasoning (Clinical Medicine) - Stages of moral reasoning categorized by particular motivations for a person's choices and actions, including in chronological order: punishment, reward, good boy/girl, authority, social contract, and ethical principle orientations.

Lear Complex (Pathology) - The libidinous fixation of a father upon a daughter.

Oedipus complex (Clinical Medicine) - Freudian concept of repressed sexual feelings that a 3-6 year old male has for the mother, as well as feelings of rivalry towards the father. Don't Confuse This With: Oedepism

Stanford-Binet Intelligence scale (Clinical Medicine) - A standardized test to measure intelligence and mental age of children compared to normal children at various ages.

Anton-Babinski syndrome (Pathology) - A psychiatric syndrome where a blind patient denies and lacks awareness of his or her own condition, and will respond with confabulations.

Electra Complex (Pathology) - Unresolved issues with father during childhood that influence a woman's interactions with men in adulthood.

Tanner Stages of Sexual Development (Clinical Medicine) - Stages of puberty that evaluate physical development by pubic hair and genitalia growth in boys and pubic hair and breast development in girls. Don't Confuse This With: Tanner growth chart

Van Gogh Syndrome (Pathology) - A factitious or malingering disorder in which the patient presents with confabulated severe illnesses dramatic and emergent in nature with the objective of being admitted. Once admitted, this patient acts violently and demands special attention.

Albatross Reaction (Pathology) - A psychological condition similar to Munchausen syndrome where the patient follows their doctor around because they believe they have a cure for everything, even for problems that the patient does not have. Don't Confuse This With: Munchausen syndrome

Alice in Wonderland syndrome (Pathology) - A psychological syndrome where the patient has a distorted view of self and surroundings. There are hallucinations and miscalculations in spatial environment, as well as a delusion of self-image. Causes may include temporal lobe epilepsy, Epstein-Barr virus and migraines. AKA Todd Syndrome. Don't Confuse This With: Hallucinogenic drug toxicity

CHAPTER 3: CARDIOVASCULAR

Note: The Cardiovascular chapter includes many high-yield eponyms & buzzwords. It would be wise to pay extra attention to the contents of this chapter.

Angle of Louis (Anatomy) - Also known as the sternal angle: located at the manubriosternal junction.

Anitschkow cells (Pathology) - Plump, activated macrophages that are a component of an Aschoff body. Seen in patients with acute Rheumatic fever. Don't Confuse This With: Aschoff body, Box-car nuclei

Aschoff bodies (Pathology) - Characteristic of acute rheumatic fever. They're discrete, inflammatory lesions specifically found in the heart, in any of the three layers. Have central zone of degenerating, hypereosinophilic matrix with an inflammatory infiltrate. Don't Confuse This With: Anitschkow cells, Box-car nuclei

Batson Plexus (Anatomy) - Vertebral venous network that provides a route for spinal and cranial metastases, often noted in regards to prostate cancer or colorectal cancer.

Berry Aneurysm (Pathology) - Congenital or acquired. Classically involves branches of the Circle of Willis. Also known as a saccular aneurysm.

Buerger disease (Pathology) - A segmental, thrombosing, acute/chronic inflammation of small and medium sized arteries. Mainly affects the tibial and radial arteries. Commonly seen in young (<35yo), heavy smokers. AKA: Thromboangitis Obliterans. Don't Confuse This With: Raynaud disease, Polyarteritis Nodosa, Horton Disease, Wegener's Granulomatosis

Bundle of His (Physiology) - Part of the conduction system of the Heart. Consists of Purkinje fibers. Arises from the atrio-ventricular node, passes and descends through the interventricular septum, and then divides to supply the right and left ventricles. Don't Confuse This With: Bundle of Kent, Bachmann bundle

Chagas' disease (Microbiology) - Is a myocarditis caused by the protozoan Trypanosoma cruzi. This parasite invades scattered myofibers, causing inflammation and that inflammation results in damage of the myocardium. Endemic in areas of South America.

Circle of Willis (Anatomy) - An intricate assembly of arteries formed at the base of the brain, supplying oxygen rich blood to brain parenchyma. Common location for cerebral aneurysms. Don't Confuse This With: Berry Aneurysm, Willis cords

Cooley anemia (Pathology) - Thalassemia Major, the most severe type of beta thalassemia.

Cor Bovinum (Pathology) - Massive left ventricular hypertrophy due to a volume overload often observed in hypertensive and ischemic heart disease. Translated, means "Cow's Heart." Don't Confuse This With: Cor Pulmonale

Cushing Triad (Clinical Medicine) - Triad of increased bradycardia, bradypnea, and hypertension. May lead to Cushing ulcers. Don't Confuse This With: Cushing Syndrome, Cushing Disease, Cushing Ulcer, Cushing Phenomenon, Addison Disease

DeBakey I, II, III Aortic Dissections (Pathology) - Classification system for aortic dissections. Type A (DeBakey I and II) are more common, involve either the ascending only or both ascending and descending aorta, and are more dangerous. Type B (DeBakey III) is a more distal lesion, beginning distal to the subclavian artery) and does not involve the ascending aorta.

Double barrel aorta (Pathology) - A radiological sign indicating aortic dissection. Don't Confuse This With: Tree Bark Aortic Intima, Machine-Like Murmur

Dressler Syndrome (Pathology) - A secondary form of pericarditis caused by an auto-immune inflammatory reaction towards myocardial neo-antigens post-myocardial infarction. Pericardial friction rub, fever, chest pain, and elevated ESR are present. Don't Confuse This With: Rheumatic heart disease, Dressler Beat

Duroziez Sign (Clinical Medicine) - A systolic and diastolic two phase murmur heard over the femoral artery with the bell of the stethoscope in patients with severe aortic regurgitation.

Eisenmenger complex (Pathology) - A defect of the interventricular septum with severe pulmonary hypertension leading to a consequent right-to-left shunt through the ventricular septal defect. Don't Confuse This With: Einthoven's triangle, Eisenmenger Syndrome

Fick Principle (Physiology) - A technique for measure cardiac output used to create the Fick equation. Assumes the total uptake of substance by the peripheral tissues is equal to the product of blood flow to the peripheral tissues and the arterio-venous concentration difference of the substance, which is oxygen. Also assumes no shunts are present.

Frank-Starling Mechanism (Physiology) - A fundamental principle stating that the greater the end-diastolic volume, the greater the stroke volume.

Henoch-Schonlein purpura (Pathology) - A systemic vasculitis characterized by immune complex deposition containing IgA in the skin and the kidney. Usually presents as a palpable purpuric rash 1-3 weeks after an upper respiratory infection. Also associated with joint and abdominal pain. Mainly occurs in small children. Don't

Confuse This With: Raynaud disease, Polyarteritis Nodosa, Horton Disease, Wegener's Granulomatosis, Waterhouse-Friderichsen Syndrome

Jones Criteria (Pathology) - A set of criteria which assist in the diagnosis of acute rheumatic heart disease in conjunction with serologic evidence of a previous streptococcal infection. Two major Jones criteria, or one of the major Jones criteria manifestations and two minor manifestations, are sufficient for diagnosis.

Kawasaki disease (Pathology) - An acute, febrile arteritis affecting medium to large sized vessels of infants and children that's usually self-limiting. Mainly involves the coronary arteries and can lead to myocardial infarction. It is the leading cause of acquired heart disease in children. Also known as mucocutaneous lymph node syndrome. Don't Confuse This With: Buerger Disease, Polyarteritis Nodosa, Horton Disease, Wegener's Granulomatosis, Reynaud Disease, Takayasu Arteritis

Keith Node (Physiology) - AKA: Sino-atrial node. This is the pacemaker of the heart.

Libman-Sacks endocarditis (Pathology) - Refers to small, sterile, granular vegetations that develop on the heart valves of patients with systemic lupus erythematosus. The lesions occur as a result of immune complex deposition and cause inflammation. Steroid use helps to prevent this from progressing. Don't Confuse This With: Lambl excrescences

Machinery-like murmurs (Pathology) - Harsh audible sound heard commonly in patients with patent ductus arteriosis (high pressure left-to-right shunts). Don't Confuse This With: Double Barrel Aorta

Prinzmetal Angina (Pathology) - A spasm of coronary vessels causing chest pain, also known as variant angina. It is chest pain that is unstable, occurring with progressively less exertion or even at rest. Occurs in people without coronary artery disease. Associated with an ST segment elevation. The cause and mechanism are not clear but the condition is associated with cocaine use.

Purkinje Fibers (Anatomy) - They are specialized myocardial fibers that can conduct electrical impulses and are located within the inner ventricular walls of the heart. Don't Confuse This With: Purkinje Cells

Raynaud disease (Pathology) - A peripheral vascular disease resulting from an exaggerated vasoconstriction of digital arteries and arterioles. Causes pallor or cyanosis mostly of the digits of the hands or feet. Also reflects an exaggeration of central and local vasomotor responses to cold or emotion. Predilection for young women. AKA: Primary Raynaud Phenomenon Don't Confuse This With: Raynaud Disease, Syndrome; Buerger disease

Raynaud phenomenon (Pathology) - Refers to vascular insufficiency of the extremities in the context of secondary arterial disease caused by SLE, scleroderma, Buerger disease, or atherosclerosis. This disorder is the "R" in C.R.E.S.T. Syndrome. AKA: Secondary Raynaud phenomenon Don't Confuse This With: Raynaud Disease, Syndrome; Buerger disease

Takayasu arteritis (Pathology) - A granulomatous vasculitis of medium to large sized arteries characterized mainly by ocular disturbances and pronounced weakening of the pulses in the upper extremities. Manifests with transmural thickening of the aortic arch and great vessels. Common in women younger than 40yo. AKA: Pulseless disease Don't Confuse This With: Buerger Disease, Polyarteritis Nodosa, Horton Disease, Wegener's Granulomatosis, Reynaud Disease, SLE, Kawasaki Disease

Tawara node (Physiology) - AKA: Atrioventricular node. Consists of modified myocardial cells located between the atria and the ventricles of the heart. Its function is to delay impulses prior to entering the Bundle of His so as to ensure the ventricles are adequately filled prior to contraction.

Tetrology of Fallot (Pathology) - The most common cause of cyanotic congenital heart disease: has four main features: Ventricular septal defect, pulmonary artery stenosis, overriding aorta, and right ventricular hypertrophy. Radiograph shows a "boot shaped heart". Don't Confuse This With: Taussig-Bing Syndrome

Wenckebach Phenomenon (Pathology) - AKA: Mobitz type I atrioventricular heart block.

Adamkiewicz, Artery of (Anatomy) – Normally arises from left posterior intercostal artery, branching from the aorta. It supplies the anterior segments of the spine. An infarct of this artery results in Anterior Spinal Cord Syndrome.

Adams-Stokes Syncope (Pathology) - Sudden loss of consciousness due to bradycardia, complete or incomplete heart block.

Austin Flint Murmur (Clinical Medicine) – Mid-diastolic low pitched rumbling murmur best heard at the cardiac apex. Associated with severe aortic regurgitation.

Bag-like heart (Pathology) - Cardiac hypertrophy and dilation of the ventricles observed with dilated cardiomyopathy. Don't Confuse This With: Box-Car Nuclei

Beck Triad (Clinical Medicine) - The triad of clinical signs including distended neck veins (Jugular Venous Distension), hypotension and distant heart sounds. Suspicious of pericardial tamponade. Don't Confuse This With: Becker Sign

Bergman Triad (Pathology) - Triad of symptoms seen with fat emboli syndrome. The symptoms include: mental status changes, petechiae (most often in the axilla and thorax) and dyspnea. Don't Confuse This With: Deep vein thrombosis, Beck's Triad, Bernheim Effect

Box-car nuclei (Pathology) - A histopathological indication of hypertensive heart disease. Myocyte diameter increases due to the addition of sarcomeres, and is associated with the presence of prominent and hyperchromatic box-car shaped nuclei. Don't Confuse This With: Bag-like heart, bread & butter pericarditis

Bread & butter pericarditis (Pathology) - Histopathological indication of fibrinous pericarditis. Don't Confuse This With: Aschoff bodies, Anitschkow cells

Bundle of Kent (Physiology) - An accessory conduction pathway between the atria and the ventricles responsible for Wolff-Parkinson-White syndrome. Don't Confuse This With: Bundle of His, Bachmann bundle

Carvallo Sign (Clinical Medicine) - Distinguishing feature of tricuspid valve regurgitation. During inspiration, there is an increase in intensity of the pansystolic murmur.

Charcot vertigo (Pathology) - Fainting as a result of cough spell, often in large male smokers, due to sustained increase in intrathoracic pressure impeding on venous return to the heart and, thereby, decreasing cardiac output. Don't Confuse This With: Charcot angina, disease, gait, joint, tubercle

Corrigan disease (Pathology) - Aortic regurgitation.

Corrigan pulse (Clinical Medicine) – AKA Water-Hammer Pulse: clinical sign that signifies a bounding or forceful pulse, associated with increased stroke volume and decreased peripheral resistance, which leads to the widened pulse pressure of aortic regurgitation.

Cushing phenomenon (Pathology) - A phenomenon, in which an increase in intracranial pressure causes occlusion of cerebral vessels and subsequent ischemia of the brain tissue, prompting a sympathetic compensatory response that leads to increased systemic blood pressure. Don't

Confuse This With: Cushing Syndrome, Cushing Disease, Cushing Ulcer, Cushing Triad, Addison Disease

Czermak vagus pressure (Physiology) - Mechanical pressure over the carotid triangle causes a decrease in heart rate and blood pressure. Not related to the vagus nerve as the name suggests. Due to stimulation of the carotid baroreceptors. Don't Confuse This With: Charcot-Weiss-Baker syndrome

Einthoven triangle (Physiology) - An imaginary equilateral triangle involving the right and left arms and either leg with the heart at its center. It represents the flow of electrical current through the body and the 3 standard limb leads of the EKG. This triangle is the basis of the modern day 12-Lead electrocardiogram.

Fish mouth valve (Pathology) - A pathological indication of rheumatic mitral stenosis in which there is thickening & calcification of valve cusps (leaflets), often with fusion of commissures and shortening & thickening of chordae tendinae Don't Confuse This With: Lidman Sachs endocarditis

Flint murmur (Pathology) - A presystolic or late diastolic murmur that's heard best over the apex of the heart. The cause is thought to be vibration of the mitral valve due to aortic regurgitation before contraction of the ventricles.

Frank Starling Law (Physiology) - With increased dilation of the heart there is an increased force of contraction.

HACEK Group (Microbiology) - Gram negative bacteria that commonly require enhanced CO2 atmosphere for culture and commonly found infecting human heart valves; Haemophilus aphrophilus, Actinobacillus actinomycetemcomitans, Cardiobacterium hominis, Eikenella corrodens, and Kingella kingae

Haldane effect (Physiology) - The phenomenon by which deoxygenated hemoglobin has a greater affinity for carbon dioxide than does oxygenated hemoglobin.

Heberden disease (Pathology) - Also known as Angina Pectoris; A clinical syndrome of chest pain caused by insufficient oxygen supply to the heart muscle. Most commonly occurs in the presence of atherosclerosis of the coronary arteries. Pain located in the precordial region and radiates to the left shoulder, arm, and hand. Don't Confuse This With: Heberden nodes

Hering Nerve (Physiology) - Afferent nerve fibers innervating the baroreceptors of the carotid sinus and the chemoreceptors in the carotid body. It increases sympathetic outflow to the heart and the blood vessels, allowing the mean arterial pressure to return to normal. Therefore an increased blood pressure would result in a diminished heart rate.

Homan's Sign (Clinical Medicine) - A sign that may indicate a diagnosis of deep venous thrombosis (DVT). It is considered positive when passive dorsiflexion of the ankle produces a sharp pain in the calf and posterior knee. It is not a reliable test due to its false positive results.

Horton Disease (Pathology) - Also known as temporal arteritis. Granulomatous chronic inflammatory disease often affecting the superficial temporal and ophthalmic arteries. Often affects elderly adults.

Kerley B Lines (Clinical Medicine) - They are horizontal lines along the lung periphery which are seen on chest x-rays and represent thickening of the interlobular septa and usually are suggestive of congestive heart disease, but can also be seen in pulmonary fibrosis, carcinomatosis. Don't Confuse This With: Kerley A lines, Kerley C lines.

Koch triangle (Anatomy) - Triangular shaped area on the right atrium of the heart composed of the tricuspid valve, sinus venosus, and Todaro tendon. Significance of this region is that it marks the site of the atrioventricular node.

Kussmaul Sign (Clinical Medicine) - Observation of increased jugular venous pressure during inspiration. Suggests impaired filling of the right ventricle due to either pericardial fluid or a poorly compliant myocardium. Don't Confuse This With: Pulsus Paradoxus

Lambl excrescences (Pathology) - Nonbacterial thrombotic endocarditis is characterized by small, sterile vegetations on cardiac valves. With time, these vegetations organize into delicate strands of fibrous tissue called Lambl excrescences. Don't Confuse This With: Lidman Sachs endocarditis, Fish-Mouth Valve

Lancisi sign (Clinical Medicine) - Large systolic jugular venous wave indicating tricuspid regurgitation.

Laplace Law (Physiology) - Physical law, useful for fluid dynamic in relatively-cylindrical structures such as blood vessels and heart chambers: *Tension = (Pressure*Radius)* divided by *Thickness of Wall*.

Le-Negre Syndrome (Pathology) - A sclerodegenerative lesion causing isolated damage of the cardiac conduction system; originates in either AV node, bundle of His, or bundle branches

Loffler Syndrome (Pathology) - Also known as simple pulmonary eosinophillia. Pulmonary infiltrates seen as transient migratory shadows on chest x-rays. Often symptomless but there may be a cough or fever. Can be a predisposing factor to restrictive cardiomyopathy.

Mobitz type I (Wenckebach) (Physiology) - Type of 2nd degree atrio-ventricular block in which there is a progressive lengthening of the PR interval until a beat is dropped, that is a P wave which is not followed by a QRS complex is observed. This condition is usually asymptomatic. Don't Confuse This With: Mobitz Type 2

Mobitz Type II (Physiology) - Type of 2nd degree atrio-ventricular block in which dropped beats occur periodically, but are NOT preceded by lengthening in the PR interval. Often observed as a 2:1 block with two P waves to on ORS complex. This condition usually results from a block within or below the bundle of His. It may progress to a 3rd degree block. Don't Confuse This With: Mobitz Type 1

Nutmeg Liver (Pathology) - A liver that has increased in both size and weight and on cut section, displays prominent passive congestion resembling the cut surface of a nutmeg. Often due to right-sided heart failure.

Osler Maneuver (Clinical Medicine) - A bedside procedure used to distinguish between true hypertension and those with pseudohypertension due to sclerosis of the large arteries. The maneuver assesses the palpability of the pulseless radial or brachial artery distal to the point of occlusion of the artery usually by cuff pressure. Don't Confuse This With: Osler's maneuver and pseudohypertension.

Pompe disease (Pathology) - An autosomal recessive, type 2 glycogen storage disease due to a deficiency in the enzyme acid maltase. The result is the deposition of glycogen in almost every organ of the body. The variant with infantile onset leads to massive cardiomegaly and premature death.

Pratt test (Clinical Medicine) - A component of physical examination of the venous system to palpate for deep venous thrombosis. It involves applying gentle pressure to the calf. A positive test will illicit pain during the application of pressure. Don't Confuse This With: Homan's test

Sturge-Weber syndrome (Pathology) - It is a rare, congenital neurological and skin disorder caused by arteriovenous malformation that occurs in the cerebrum. Patients tend to present with portwine nevi on the scalp along with ipsilateral leptomeningeal angioma. Don't Confuse This With: Henoch-Schonlein Purpura

Tree bark appearance of the aortic intima (Pathology) - Observed in the tertiary stage of syphilis due to contraction of the connective tissue of the walls of the aorta, with degeneration of the aortic media. Don't Confuse This With: Double Barrel Aorta

Trendelenburg test (Clinical Medicine) - Test used to examine a patient for venous insufficiency of the lower extremities. The leg is raised to 90 degrees and held for 60 seconds. A tourniquet is then tied, the patient is asked to stand and the physician must observe for rapid filling. The tourniquet is removed and rapid venous filling is observed again. Don't Confuse This With: Trendelenburg Gait, Sign

Valsalva Maneuver (Clinical Medicine) - Is performed by forcible exhaling air against a closed glottis. An abnormal response of blood pressure and heart rate during this test can indicate heart abnormalities such as aortic stenosis, tricuspid regurgitation, etc. It is also used to arrest episodes of supraventricular tachycardia.

Van Lohuizen Syndrome (Pathology) - Cutaneous malformation of the capillary-venous system causing a marbled appearance.

Water-Hammer Pulse (Pathology) - Clinical sign that signifies a bounding or forceful pulse. Associated with increased stroke volume and decrease in the peripheral resistance that leads to the widened pulse pressure of aortic regurgitation.

Wenckebach Heart (Pathology) - A heart that is located in the middle of the thorax and is smaller in size than normal.

Adson test (Clinical Medicine) - A clinical finding of Thoracic outlet syndrome. Pulse disappears when patient stares in the direction of their outstretched abducted upper limb.

Allen test (Clinical Medicine) - test commonly used to demonstrate patent ulnar and radial arteries as well as an intact superficial palmar arch. Don't Confuse This With: Allen's Sign

Aschner-Dagnini test (Clinical Medicine) - An oculocardial reflex where applying pressure to the eyeball or carotid sinus can decrease the pulse rate, thereby decrease anginal pain. It is sometimes used during supraventricular tachycardia.

Auenbrugger Sign (Clinical Medicine) - an epigastric bulge caused by a very large pericardial effusion.

Barlow disease (Pathology) - Mitral valve prolapse.

Barth Syndrome (Pathology) - X linked recessive trait characterized by distortion of metabolism, delayed motor skills, stamina deficiency, hypotonia, delayed growth, chronic fatigue, and dilated cardiomyopathy.

Becker Sign (Clinical Medicine) - Visible pulsations of the retinal arteriole observed in aortic regurgitation. Don't Confuse This With: Water-Hammer Pulse, Beck's Triad

Bernheim Effect (Pathology) - Right ventricular failure caused by aortic stenosis-induced hypertrophy of the interventricular septum and its bulging into the right ventricle, compromising ventricular filling. Don't Confuse This With: Bergman Triad

Bernheim Effect - Reverse (Pathology) - Seen in cardiac tamponade and pulmonary embolism where right ventricular dysfunction with associated leftward bulging of the interventricular septum causes interference with left ventricular filling.

Blue Baby syndrome (Pathology) - Layman term used to describe newborn babies with cyanotic conditions including congenital defects of the heart and / or respiratory distress syndrome.

Button-hole stenosis (Pathology) - see Fish-Mouth Valve. Don't Confuse This With: Lidman Sachs endocarditis

Charcot-Weiss-Baker syndrome (Pathology) - Strong pressure over the bifurcation of the carotid arteries causes excitation of the carotid baroreceptors. This leads to transient attacks of syncope, marked decrease in heart rate and blood pressure, and loss of consciousness. More common in men over 45yo. Don't Confuse This With: Czermak vagus pressure

Churg-Strauss Syndrome (Pathology) - An allergic auto-immune vasculitis affecting medium to small sized vessels. This condition involves blood vessels of the lungs, gastrointestinal system and peripheral nerves. Was once considered a type of polyarteritis nodosa. Don't Confuse This With: Buerger Disease, Polyarteritis Nodosa

Corvisart facies (Clinical Medicine) - Cyanotic face with puffy eyelids seen in cardiac insufficiency or aortic regurgitation.

Dohle-Heller Syndrome (Pathology) - Inflammation of the aorta secondary to a syphilitic infection. Common complications of this condition are aortic valve insufficiency, coronary stenosis and aortic aneurysm.

Epstein syndrome (Pathology) - A very rare congenital condition with downward displacement of the tricuspid valve from the annulus fibrosis possibly leading to cardiac arrhythmias, fatigue, dyspnea, cyanosis, and sudden death.

Eisenmenger Syndrome (Pathology) - A congenital, progressive cardiac failure due to Eisenmenger Complex. Don't Confuse This With: Eisenmenger Complex

Faget Sign (Clinical Medicine) - Occurring with yellow fever, Colorado tick fever or infection caused by tularemia, brucellosis, Legionella pneumonia, Mycoplasma pneumonia, resulting in manifestation of a slow pulse accompanied by fever.

Friedel Pick Disease (Pathology) - Constrictive pericarditis due to tuberculosis, rheumatic fever, or pneumococcal infection; manifests mostly in childhood and is associated with secondary liver cirrhosis, ascites, and fibrosis. Don't Confuse This With: Niemann-Pick Disease

Gallavardin phenomenon (Clinical Medicine) - Dissociation of noisy and musical elements of aortic stenosis ejection murmurs. The musical element is heard best at the left sternal boarder and apex; lower left sternal edge presents the noisy element.

Graham Steell murmur (Clinical Medicine) - An early diastolic murmur of pulmonary regurgitation secondary to pulmonary hypertension. Also known as Steell's murmur.

Grocco sign (Clinical Medicine) - An acute dilation of the heart following a muscular effort. Usually seen in patients with Graves disease.

Heubner Disease (Pathology) - Endarteritis obliterans specifically seen in brain's of patients with syphilis.

Hines' Test (aka Hines-Brown Test) (Clinical Medicine) - A test in which the cardiovascular system is challenged by immersing one hand in ice cold water for 2 or more minutes in order to detect latent states of hypertension.

Hippocratic fingers (Pathology) - Clubbing of the fingers, which is often observed in a number of condition of the heart and lungs. Don't Confuse This With: Hippocratic Oath

Holmes Heart (Pathology) - A condition in which there is a single primitive ventricle with normally related great vessels.

Jaccoud Sign (Clinical Medicine) - Prominence of the aorta in the supersternal notch, usually an indication of leukemia.

Janeway lesions (Clinical Medicine) - Painless, small, erythematous palmar macular lesions often observed in patients with subacute infective endocarditis. Don't Confuse This With: Roth Spots, Osler Nodes

Keshan Disease (Pathology) - Potentially fatal form of cardiomyopathy caused by a deficiency of selenium, an essential mineral. More commonly observed in China.

Kippel disease (Pathology) - A condition occurring in arthritis, in which there is a generalized weakness or pseudoparalysis. Associated with intracranial atheromas.

Kommerell diverticulum (Pathology) - A congenital anomaly in which the left subclavian artery arises from this diverticulum on the aortic arch. The artery passes behind the esophagus and to the left arm.

Korotkoff test (Clinical Medicine) - A test for collateral circulation. The artery above the aneurysm is compressed and at the same time, the blood pressure in the distal circulation is estimated. If the pressure is significantly high, the collateral circulation is said to be good.

Landolfi Sign (Clinical Medicine) - Systolic contraction and diastolic dilation of the pupil; seen in patients suffering from aortic insufficiency.

Leriche Syndrome (Pathology) - Aortoiliac occlusive disease; causes distal ischemic symptoms, pulselessness, impotence, atrophy of the buttocks. Don't Confuse This With: Leriche Operation

Liebermeister Rule (Physiology) - A rule describing the relationship between pulse rate and body temperature in patients with adult febrile tachycardia. Approximatey 8 pulse beats corresponds to a 1°C increase in temperature.

Loeffler endomyocarditis (Pathology) - A form of restrictive cardiomyopathy. Causes endocardial fibrosis, typically with large mural thrombi. No geographic restrictions. Associated with peripheral hypereosinophilia. Much of the endocardial damage is thought to be caused by release of Major Basic Protein. Don't Confuse This With: Endomyocardial fibrosis, Lidman-Sachs Endocarditis, Other Endocarditis

Ludwig Ganglion (Physiology) - A ganglion, or parasympathetic nerve cell bundle in the interarterial septum. Don't Confuse This With: Ludwig Angle

Lutembacher syndrome (Pathology) - A very rare form of heart disease. Characterized by atrial septal defect, mitral stenosis, dilation and hypertrophy of right side of heart. Usually congenital but may be acquired via rheumatic fever. Don't Confuse This With: Cossio syndrome

Monckeberg sclerosis (Pathology) - Calcific deposits in muscular arteries, usually in people over the age of 50 years-old. It is radiographically visible and often palpable. However, it does not occlude the lumen and therefore, carries little clinical significance. Don't Confuse This With: Buerger Disease, Polyarteritis Nodosa, Horton Disease, Wegener's Granulomatosis

Muller Sign (Clinical Medicine) - Sign characteristic of aortic valve regurgitation in which the uvula rhythmically pulsates with the contraction of the heart. Don't Confuse This With: Muller Law

Neubauer artery (Anatomy) - Synonym for thyroid ima artery. Don't Confuse This With: Thyroid ima artery

Osborn waves (Pathology) - Term used to describe an extra dome shaped deflection found on a 12-Lead EKG at the R-ST junction. Commonly seen in patients experiencing hypothermia. Don't Confuse This With: Heberden Disease

Pardee waves (Pathology) - Waves that show up as deep symmetrically inverted T waves on the EKG at times of myocardial infarction or ischemic heart disease.

Pickwickian syndrome (Pathology) - A disorder affecting chest movement that predisposes patients to cor pulmonale. It is characterized by obstructive apnea in moderately to severely obese people, alveolar hypoventilation, right sided heart failure (cor pulmonale), cyanosis of the extremities and lips, secondary polycythemia, reddish complexion, prolonged drowsiness.

Roth Spot (Pathology) - Often seen in retinal hemorrhagic conditions where there is a round, white retinal spot surrounded by areas of hemorrhages close to the optic disk. Typically seen in endocarditis.

Stokes syndrome (Pathology) - see Adams-Stokes Syncope

Traube sign / phenomenon (Clinical Medicine) - Upon auscultation, a double "pistol shot" sound heard over the femoral artery in conditions involving aortic insufficiency.

Wolff-Parkinson-White syndrome (Pathology) - Is a syndrome characterized by a pre-excitation of the ventricles due to an accessory pathway known as the bundle of Kent. These individuals are at high risk for tachyarrhythmia and sudden death. EKG shows delta-wave pattern in limb leads.

Abrams' heart reflex I (Pathology) - Contraction of myocardium with reduction in area of cardiac dullness upon irritation of skin in the precordial region. Most pronounced in children and in adults who have poorly developed muscles and fatty upholster. Don't Confuse This With: Abrams heart reflex II

Abrams' heart reflex II (Pathology) - A cutivisceral reflex in patients with angina pectoris. The chest pain is relieved and pain area reduced if the skin overlying the region of irradiating pain is irritated, followed by Abrams' heart reflex I. Don't Confuse This With: Abrams heart reflex I

Albini nodules (Pathology) - Small fibrous nodules located along the margins of mitral and tricuspid valves. Sometimes seen in neonates; represent fetal tissue rests.

Anrep effect (Pathology) - A transient positive inotropic effect and regulatory mechanism of the heart in response to increased afterload. Also known as homeometric autoregulation. Functions independently of muscle length. Related to recovery from transient subendocardial ischemia.

Austrian Triad (Clinical Medicine) - Clinical triad of meningitis, endocarditis and pneumococcal pneumonia.

Bachmann bundle (Physiology) - One of the four conduction tracts that make up the atrial conduction tract transmitting electrical impulses from the SA node to the rest of the heart. Don't Confuse This With: Bundle of Kent, Bundle of His

Bancroft sign (Clinical Medicine) - common test used to determine the presence of deep venous thrombosis.

Bjork-Shiley valve (Clinical Medicine) - single tilting disk prosthetic mechanical heart valve. Has been used to replaced aortic and mitral valves.

Bland-White-Garland syndrome (Pathology) - Characterized by left ventricular failure, congenital or occurring shortly after birth. There is a malformation in which the left coronary artery arises from the pulmonary artery and not from the aorta. The symptoms include failure to thrive, dyspnea, tachypnea, precordial pain, pallor, and crying after feeding.

Bradbury-Eggleston syndrome (Pathology) - A degenerative, autonomic disorder characterized by abnormally low blood pressure while in the standing position.

Branham sign (Clinical Medicine) - compression of the AV fistula causing bradycardia. It is also known as Nicoladoni sign.

Buerger Sign (Clinical Medicine) - Sign which demonstrates peripheral vascular disease; red foot becomes pale with elevation.

Charcot angina (Pathology) - Insufficiency of blood flow in the whole body resulting in gait disturbances, pain, discomfort, cramps. Don't Confuse This With: Charcot disease, gait, joint, tubercle, vertigo

Corkscrew vessels (Clinical Medicine) - Blood vessels that double back on themselves; may indicate early invasive cervical cancer.

Crescendo Angina (Pathology) - Angina pectoris that occurs with increasing intensity, duration and/or frequency.

Da Costa Syndrome (Pathology) - A syndrome that has symptoms similar to heart disease. However, upon physical exam, the patient does not elicit any problems. It is suggested to be caused by anxiety disorder and stress. This syndrome is also known as Soldier's Heart.

Damus-Kaye-Stansel procedure (Clinical Medicine) - It is an operative procedure that is used to repair various heart abnormalities including congenital transposition of the great vessels.

De Musset sign (Clinical Medicine) - Shaking of the head and body that occurs in rhythm with beats of the heart and it is observed in people with aortic regurgitation.

Dressler Beat (Clinical Medicine) - fusion beat observe din ventricular tachycardia producing a narrow QRS complex on ECG. Don't Confuse This With: Dressler Syndrome

Fahr syndrome (Pathology) - Rare, idiopathic disease resulting in areas of calcifications of small brain vessels. Occurs mostly during the middle age and manifests as mental retardation, dystonic movements, and athetosis.

Fay Sign (Clinical Medicine) - Pressure along the carotid nerve causing pain to be distributed to the distal branches of the external carotid nerve to the jaw, template and the ear. Seen in carotid arteritis.

Flack test (Clinical Medicine) - AKA Valsalva maneuver.

Gairdner disease (Pathology) - Episodic attacks of cardiac distress with apprehension; synonymous to angina pectoris.

Gärtner vein phenomenon (Clinical Medicine) - The degree of fullness of the arm veins as the arm is raised above the heart and the point at which the veins collapse helps to indicate right atrial pressure. Don't Confuse This With: Gardner Syndrome

Gerbode defect (Pathology) - Defect in the interventricular septum associated with communication of the right atrium with the left ventricle.

Gerhardt Sign (Clinical Medicine) - Pulsation of the spleen in the presence of splenomegaly observed in aortic regurgitation. Also known as Sailor's sign.

Gibson murmur (Clinical Medicine) - This is the name that is given to the "machinery-like" murmur of patent ductus arteriosus.

Great vein of Galen (Anatomy) - Large unpaired vein formed by the junction of the two internal cerebral veins near the third ventricle. Also known as the great cerebral vein. Don't Confuse This With: Canal of Guyon

Guyon Sign (Clinical Medicine) - To distinguish the internal carotid artery from the external carotid, look for hypoglossal nerve that lies on the external carotid. Don't Confuse This With: Canal of Guyon

Hollenhorst plaques (Pathology) - Cholesterol emboli that are found in the arterioles of the retina.

Lev disease (Pathology) - An acquired complete heart block that results due to idiopathic calcification and fibrosis of the signal conduction system of the heart. Also known as Lenegre-Lev syndrome. May lead to Stokes-Adams Attacks.

Louvel sign (Clinical Medicine) - Venous pain that is induced during coughing and that is prevented by pressing over the proximal end of the vein. Observed in deep vein thrombosis.

Milroy disease (Pathology) - A form of primary, chronic hereditary lymphedema of the limbs, leading to pitting and swelling of the feet and ankles. Due to an anatomically abnormal lymphatic system. Don't Confuse This With: Meige Disease, Elephantitis

Morgagni Disease (Pathology) - aka Adams-Stokes Syndrome. Don't Confuse This With: Morgagni Glands, Syndrome, Globules

Palla sign (Clinical Medicine) - Enlargement of the right descending coronary artery that can occur with pulmonary embolism

Sinuses of Valsalva (Anatomy) - Three dilations in the wall of the ascending aorta just above the cusps of the aortic valve. The left aortic sinus gives ruse to the left coronary artery, the right aortic sinus gives rise to the right coronary artery and no vessels typically arise from the posterior aortic sinus.

Thebesian, Valve of (Physiology) - The valve of the coronary sinus, located at the entrance to the right atrium. Don't Confuse This With: Thebesian, Vein of

Wardrop Method (Clinical Medicine) - procedure to treat an aneurysm by ligating artery at some distance beyond the sac to leave arterial branches between sac and ligature.

Achenbach Syndrome (Pathology) - A disorder of unknown etiology that affects both men and women and involves a coin-sized hematoma on the palm of the hand. The hematoma is painful and edematous, particularly after a temperature change. Don't Confuse This With: Trauma

Alfidi Syndrome (Pathology) - Hypertension resulting from occlusion of the celiac axis, leading to diversion of collateral blood flow from the right renal artery. Don't Confuse This With: Ischemic bowel disease

Anel operation (Clinical Medicine) - A surgical procedure involving the ligation of an artery proximal to an aneurysm.

Antopol disease (Pathology) - Abnormal glycogen deposits in the heart and systemic muscles cause cardiomegaly and muscle weakness.

Batista procedure (Clinical Medicine) - Partial left ventriculectomy, performed as a treatment for heart failure.

Beau syndrome (Pathology) - Characterized by myocardial insufficiency due to an inability to complete systole; mainly involves ventricles.

Brechenmacher fibers (Physiology) - Tracts within the heart connecting the atrium to the bundle of His

Chiari net (Pathology) - Abnormal fibrous strands in the right atrium.

Cogan syndrome (Pathology) - Vasculitis most commonly appearing in third decade of life and affecting CNS vessels, most commonly with eye and ear involvement and can be associated with aortitis.

Collett-Edwards classification (Clinical Medicine) - System of classification for congenital heart defects.

Concato disease (Pathology) - Constrictive pericarditis with polyserositis.

Cossio-Perianes Operation (Clinical Medicine) - A surgical procedure whereby the inferior vena cava is ligated as treatment for patients with decompensated heart disease.

Cossio syndrome (Pathology) - A congenital malformation of the heart characterized by atrial septal defect and mitral valve stenosis, resulting in a left-to-right shunt. Don't Confuse This With: Lutembacher syndrome

Coumel tachycardia (Pathology) - Persistent junctional reciprocating tachycardia involving posterograde conduction.

Eberth Lines (Microbiology) - Lines that appear between myocytes when stained with silver nitrate.

Ehret phenomenon (Clinical Medicine) - A throb that is felt by the finger on the brachial artery during blood pressure measurement. Indicates the diastolic pressure.

Gronblad-Strandberg syndrome (Pathology) - A rare genetic disease with degenerated elastic fibers in the skin, blood vessels and heart as a result of calcification. Cardiovascular complications present as absence of pulse in arms and legs, intermittent claudication, hypertension, angina pectoris, and stenosis of the celiac artery.

Halasz syndrome (Pathology) - Multiple congenital abnormalities of the thorax. Characterized by hypoplasia of the right lung, dextroposition of the heart, and abnormal pulmonary venous return. Principle radiological sign is an arc-like shadow, resembling a Turkish sword.

Hamman sign (Clinical Medicine) - A crunching, rasping sound that's synchronous with the heartbeat heard in patient's with spontaneous mediastinal emphysema.

Hegglin syndrome (Pathology) - Is an energy-dynamic cardiac insufficiency often seen during diabetic coma or other significant metabolic disturbance. S2 is heard soon after S1, before its corresponding T-wave, and the length of QT interval is increased.

Hess Test (Clinical Medicine) - See Rumpel-Leede Sign.

Klinger syndrome (Pathology) - See Wegener granulomatosis.

Koltipin syndrome (Pathology) - Cardiac symptoms in patient's with Scarlet fever, characterized by tachycardia, decreased blood pressure, unchangeable border of the heart, and sweating.

Korotkov sounds (Physiology) - Circulatory sounds auscultated upon checking the blood pressure when the pressure over the artery is lower than systolic pressure because of the sphygmomanometer cuff. The sound is produced by the sudden distension of the vessel. Don't Confuse This With: Korotkoff test

Laënnec thrombus (Pathology) - A globular, antenatal thrombus located in the heart.

Langendorff Method (Physiology) - Method of perfusing isolated mammalian heart by carrying fluid under pressure into coronary system via the sectioned aorta

Langendorff apparatus (Physiology) - Apparatus for the artificial perfusion of an excised heart. It is a very important method for the pharmacological and physiological research of the heart, as well as cardiac surgery and cardiac preservation.

Leriche Operation (Clinical Medicine) - Periarterial sympathectomy Don't Confuse This With: Leriche Syndrome

Lillehei-Nakib toroidal valve (Pathology) - A mechanical heart valve developed in the 1960's mainly for the purpose of replacing the mitral valve. With mechanical heart valves, patients are at risk of developing infective endocarditis along the suture line and perivalvular tissue and may cause the valve to detach. Don't Confuse This With: Bioprosthetic valves

Luciani periods (Physiology) - Term used to describe the periodic cardiac rhythm or cardiac group beating. Characterized by three distinct phenomena, which occur prior to cardiac exhaustion: access, periodic rhythm, and crisis. Don't Confuse This With: Mobitz Type 1 or 2

Mannkopf Sign (Clinical Medicine) - Increased pulse rate elicited by applied pressure to a painful spot on the body.

Nick procedure (Clinical Medicine) - A surgical procedure involving the enlargement of the aortic annulus by incising the noncoronary sinus and the roof of the left atrium.

Norwood operation (Clinical Medicine) - Surgery performed in infants with subaortic stenosis and tricuspid atresia. Involves reconstructing the aorta using the pulmonary artery.

Ortner Syndrome (Pathology) - Rare condition where impingement of recurrent laryngeal nerve by an enlarged left atrium causes a horse voice.

Pott aneurysm (Pathology) - An aneurysm of the venous system in which an artery drains directly into a vein causing distention and tortuosity. Don't Confuse This With: Pott Disease

Retzius, Veins of (Anatomy) - Portacaval anastomoses of small veins that connect the retroperitoneal organs to venous branches of the inferior vena cava. Retzius venous dilation attributed to portal hypertension.

Roger Disease (Pathology) - Inborn, asymptomatic ventricular septal defect 0.5 cm or smaller. Loud murmur can be present. Don't Confuse This With: Roberts Disease

Rumpel-Leede Sign (Clinical Medicine) - Test used to determine the integrity of capillaries by raising the venous pressure in the forearm with a BP cuff and examining the skin for petechiae. Synonymous with Hess Test.

Sappey, Veins of (Anatomy) - AKA paraumbilical veins of the portal venous system. Veins connecting azygos vein to the epigastric and internal mammary veins. Can become dilated with portal hypertension. Don't Confuse This With: Sappey, Plexus of

Singleton-Merten syndrome (Pathology) - A very rare disorder characterized by calcification of the aortic arch along with hypertrophy of the heart and dental abnormalities. An autosomal dominant inheritance has been suggested.

Spens Syndrome (Pathology) - see Adams-Stokes Syncope.

Spider cells (Pathology) - Immature variant of muscle cells. They are large, round or polygonal cells containing numerous glycogen-laden vacuoles that are separated by strands of cytoplasm running from the plasma membrane to the centrally located nucleus. Characteristically seen rhabdomyosarcomas of the heart.

Taussig-Bing syndrome (Pathology) - A rare congenital abnormality in which the aorta arises from the right ventricle and the pulmonary artery arises from both ventricles. Also occurs in association with a large ventricular septal defect, right ventricular hypertrophy, and cardiomegaly. Don't Confuse This With: Tetrology of Fallot

Thebesian, Veins of (Anatomy) - Small veins that drain the myocardium to the right atrium. Don't Confuse This With: Thebesian, Valve of

Todaro tendon (Anatomy) - A tendon that is located in the right atrium of the heart muscle, connecting the atrial fibrous trigone to the Eustachian valve of the inferior vena cava.

Uhl Syndrome (Pathology) - Rare syndrome in which right ventricular myocardium does not develop. The right ventricle is hypocontractile, thin, and fibrous. This condition may lead to cyanosis, cardiac failure, or sudden death in infancy.

Westberg space (Anatomy) - Space around origin of the aorta, invested with pericardium.

CHAPTER 4: EMBRYOLOGY & DEVELOPMENT

Potter Sequence (Pathology) - Oligohydramnios due to renal agenesis or amniotic fluid leak causing pulmonary hypoplasia, amnion nodosum, and fetal compression Don't Confuse This With: Potter Syndrome, Pott Disease

Simian Crease (Clinical Medicine) - Clinical sign found in hands relating to Down syndrome (Trisomy 21).

Tourette Syndrome (Pathology) - A childhood disorder characterized by involuntary motor and vocal tics as well as vocalized profanities that are present longer than a year and begin before the age of 18. Don't Confuse This With: Tourette disease

Edwards syndrome (Pathology) - Congenital disorder with trisomy 18; life expectancy is less than one year with severe mental retardation; prominent occiput, low-set ears, congenital heart defects and Rocker-bottom feet.

Fragile-X (Biochemistry) - An X-linked recessive disease where methylation and expression of FMR1 gene is interrupted; associated with chromosomal breakage and is second most common genetic mental retardation cause; triplet repeat disorder.

Landau Reflex (Physiology) - Infancy reflex (3 mo. - 2 yr.): lifting the thorax should induce extension of neck, spine and limbs. Don't Confuse This With: Landau-Kleffner Syndrome

Patau syndrome (Genetics) - Congenital disorder with trisomy 13; life expectancy is less than one year with severe mental retardation, cleft lip/palate, polydactyl, heart defects and rocker-bottom feet.

Potter Syndrome (Pathology) - Bilateral renal agenesis due to malformation of the ureteric bud, which leads to limb and facial deformities (Potter facies), as well as pulmonary hypoplasia which leads to death due to respiratory failure Don't Confuse This With: Potter Sequence, Pott Disease

Treacher Collins Syndrome (Pathology) - An autosomal dominant disorder in which mandibulofacial dysostosis is present with structures derived from the first pharyngeal arch showing bone abnormalities; characterized by "fish-like" face with underdeveloped zygomatic bones, downward sloping palpebral fissures, small mandible, and malformed ears.

Turner Syndrome (Pathology) - This is a genetic disorder that occurs in females and the genotype is 45, X. The typical clinical features are short stature, webbing of the neck, widely spaced nipples on the chest, lymphedema of the hands and feet, horseshoe kidney, diabetes, bicuspid aortic valve, and coarctation of the aorta. Unlike in Kleinfelter syndrome, this syndrome is responsible for primary hypogonadism in females. Don't Confuse This With: Klinefelter Syndrome

Wharton Jelly (Anatomy) - Mucous connective tissue of umbilical cord.

Clifford disease (Pathology) - Prolonged gestation causes decreased alertness, increased respiratory distress, and low birth weight in infants.

Francois' syndrome (Pathology) - Multiple congenital abnormalities of unknown etiology affecting both sexes, characterized by abnormally shaped skull, dwarfism, abnormalities in the facial features, atrophy of the skin, skeletal abnormalities, mental retardation and congenital cataracts.

Hallermann syndrome (Pathology) - A congenital abnormality characterized by a proportionate dwarfism, abnormal shaped skull, bird-like face with a beaked nose and small mandible, atrophy of the skin and mental retardation.

Rocker-bottom feet (Biochemistry) - Clinical sign found in feet relating to Patau syndrome (Trisomy 13) and Edwards' syndrome (Trisomy 18).

Rubinstein-Taybi syndrome (Genetics) - An X linked recessive disease characterized by features such as small trunk, prominent forehead, depressed nasal bridge, cleft soft palate, small jaw, and impaired hearing.

Taybi-Linder syndrome (Pathology) - Intrauterine growth retardation probably due to autosomal recessive inheritance; characterized by dwarfism, low birth weight, bone malformation, and cerebral abnormalities.

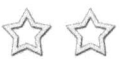

Hall-Pallister Syndrome (Pathology) - An extremely rare, embryological malformation characterized by hamartoma in hypothalamic tract, hypopituitarism, imperforate anus and polydactyl.

Andermann syndrome (Pathology) - Congenital absence of the corpus callosum.

CHARGE complex (Pathology) - Diagnosed in infants with four of seven components: Coloboma, Heart defects, Atresia of nasal choanae, Retarded growth, Genitalia hypoplasia, Ear abnormalities and/or deafness.

Werdnig-Hoffmann disease (Genetics) - Autosomal recessive disease characterized by a "floppy baby," tongue fasciculations, and death by the age of 7 months.

Chapter 5: Endocrine

Addison Disease (Pathology) - This is a rare disorder that is due to a progressive destruction of the adrenal cortex of the adrenal gland leading to a deficiency of mineralocorticoids, glucocorticoids and adrenal androgens. Destruction may be due to an autoimmune disease, tuberculosis, AIDS or various cancers. For symptoms to manifest, at least 90% of the cortex needs to be destroyed. Pigmentation of the skin may also occur due to the increased amount of ACTH and MSH, which stimulates melanocytes. Without hormone replacement, death may ensue. Don't Confuse This With: Addison Anemia, melanoderma; Conn Syndrome; Cushing Syndrome; Phenomenon, Disease, Ulcer, Triad

Cushing Syndrome (Pathology) - Just like Cushing Disease, this syndrome is the result of elevated levels of cortisol in the blood, but the cause is not restricted to an ACTH-secreting pituitary adenoma. The most common reason is administration of exogenous glucocorticoids through medication. Other, less common reasons include primary adrenocortical neoplasia, also known as ACTH-independent Cushing syndrome, and ectopic secretion of ACTH from other non-endocrine neoplasms. Also, if the cause is a primary adrenocortical neoplasia, the skin does not appear tanned, because the excess cortisol is inhibiting the production of ACTH, thus reducing the melanocyte stimulation by MSH. Don't Confuse This With: Cushing Disease, Phenomenon, Triad, Ulcer; Addison Disease; Conn Syndrome

Cushing Disease (Pathology) - This is a hypercortisolemia disorder induced by an ACTH-secreting pituitary adenoma and is more common in women than in men. Other causes of hypercortisolemia result in Cushing Syndrome. Classic symptoms of this disorder include rapid weight gain, moon face, a buffalo hump on the back of the neck, thinning of skin, striae, and tanned appearing skin. Excess cortisol also suppresses the immune system; hence these patients are more susceptible to infection. Treatment is surgical excision of the pituitary adenoma. Don't Confuse This With: Cushing Syndrome, Cushing Phenomenon, Cushing Ulcer, Cushing Triad, Addison Disease, Conn Syndrome

Grave Disease (Pathology) - This is the most common cause of hyperthyroidism in females. This is an autoimmune disorder with the most common antibody being directed toward the TSH receptor on the thyroid follicular cells. The characteristic findings in Grave's disease include thyrotoxicosis, exophthalmos, and pretibial myxedema. The thyrotoxicosis is caused by the stimulation of the thyroid gland with the anti-TSH receptor antibody, the exophthalmos is caused by the deposition of retro-orbital connective tissue and the weakening of the extraocular muscles, and pretibial myxedema is a non-pitting edema. To help distinguish from other forms of the hyperthyroidism, the laboratory findings in this condition include increased serum free T4 and T3 and decreased serum TSH levels. Also, since the thyroid is being constantly stimulated, the radioactive scan would demonstrate a diffuse uptake of iodine by the follicular cells. This condition may be treated with drugs that counteract the excess thyroid hormone or surgical removal of the gland itself followed by the supplementation of the missing thyroid hormone. Don't Confuse This With: Hashimoto's thyroditis

Hashimoto Thyroditis (Pathology) - this is the most common cause for hypothyroidism. This disease is a result of an autoimmune disease that targets the thyrocytes and causes their destruction. As a result, the thyroid gland will appear fibrosed with mononuclear cell infiltrate. Some of the characteristic findings that are visible on the histological slide include the germinal centers as a result of the infiltration and the hurthle, or oxyphil, cells that are a metaplastic response to the injury. Although this condition manifests itself as a hypothyroid condition, in the beginning there is a transient elevation in serum thyroid hormone. This is a result of the transient destruction of the thyroid follicular cells due to the auto antibodies, which release their stored T3 and T4 hormones. This condition is referred to as Hashitoxicosis. However, as the disease progresses, the T3 and T4 levels drop and the TSH levels increase due to the lack of inhibition. These laboratory finding are the opposite of what would be expected from someone with Grave's Disease. Treatment for this condition is to simply replace the thyroid hormone.   Don't Confuse This With: Grave's Disease

Waterhouse-Friderichsen syndrome (Pathology) - Infection of adrenal glands due to systemic spread of N. meningitidis; characterized by disseminated intravascular coagulation (DIC), purpura, shock, meningococcemia. Don't Confuse This With: Disseminated intravascular coagulation (DIC); Henoch–Schönlein purpura

Zollinger-Ellison Syndrome (Pathology) - Syndrome characterized by a duodenal or pancreatic gastrinoma with associated hypergastrinemia. Altered gastrin levels lead to an increase in gastric acid secretion and chronic peptic ulcers. This syndrome is part of Multiple Endocrine Neoplasia 1 (MEN1). Don't Confuse This With: Zollner Lines

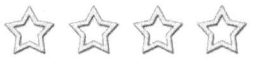

Conn Syndrome (Pathology) - Also known as primary hyperaldosteronism. This syndrome results from an aldosterone-secreting adenoma of the adrenal gland, which result in salt and water retention, and hypertension. Don't Confuse This With: Cushing Syndrome, Cushing Phenomenon, Cushing Disease, Cushing Ulcer, Cushing Triad, Addison Disease, Conn Syndrome

Forbes-Albright syndrome (Pathology) - Amenorrhea-galactorrhea syndrome in the presence of pituitary prolactin producing adenoma.

Hurthle cell (Pathology) - Specialized epithelial cells with eosinophilic granular cytoplasm found in Hashimoto thyroditis and thyroid adenomas. The normal epithelial cells of the thyroid gland are low cuboidal in shape. With constant injury, however, these cells undergo a metaplastic response and become Hurthle cells.

Klinefelter Syndrome (Pathology) - A developmental genetic disorder with genotype 47, XXY. The most common manifestation of this condition is hypogonadism that results in the testes being as small as 2 cm, gynecomastia, reduced facial and pubic hair, mild mental retardation, and diabetes. Don't Confuse This With: Turner Syndrome

Sheehan Syndrome (Pathology) - Also known as Postpartum hypopituitarism or postpartum pituitary necrosis. This condition results in reduced function of the pituitary gland due to blood loss during pregnancy and/or labor. During pregnancy, the number of prolactin secreting cells increases dramatically in the anterior pituitary, but this gland enlargement does not undergo additional vascularization so the gland is more susceptible to ischemic injury. This necrosis of the anterior pituitary can cause a variety of problems, including: pituitary dwarfism, amenorrhea, infertility, impotence, and pallor (because MSH is not being produced). Don't Confuse This With: Prolactinoma

Dalrymple Sign (Clinical Medicine) - Atypical widening of the palpebral fissure causing retraction of the upper eyelid which is seen in Grave's disease.

De Quervain thyroiditis (Pathology) - Also known as Subacute Granulomatous Thyroiditis. Although the exact etiology of this condition is unknown, it is postulated that it is due to a prior viral infection. Don't Confuse This With: subacute lymphocytic thyroiditis, Hashimoto's thyroiditis, Riedel thyroiditis, de Quervain tenosynovitis

Fibiger-Debré von Gierke syndrome (Pathology) - Inborn error of metabolism characterized by a deficiency of enzymes used in production of adrenocorticosteroid hormones, resulting in salt loss.

Kallmann Syndrome (Pathology) - Disorder of hypothalamic function and decreased gonadotropic activity. Characterized by hypogonadism, eunuchoidism and anosmia.

Achard-Thiers Syndrome (Pathology) - A condition in post-menopausal women that combines the symptoms of Cushing's Syndrome and androgenital syndrome. Women present with hirsutism, menstrual disorders, diabetes mellitus, obesity, genital hyperplasia, and an adenoma of the adrenal cortex. Don't Confuse This With: Cushing's Syndrome, androgenital syndrome

Laron-type Dwarfism (Pathology) - Deficiency of IGF-1 (insulin-like growth factor) or abnormalities of its receptor resulting in dwarfism.

Plummer Syndrome (Pathology) - This condition is common in women over the age of 60 and results in patients that have had a goiter for a long time. Usually a goiter is nonfunctional and its most common clinical feature is a mass effect on the surrounding neck structures. For example, it may cause dysphagia, compression of vessels and nerves, and obstruction of the airways. In this syndrome, a nodule may develop on the goiter that may be hyperfunctional and cause the secretion of excessive amounts of thyroid hormone. As a result, this condition may resemble Grave's disease. However, unlike Grave's

Disease, there are no peripheral signs of pretibial myxedema and exophthalmos.

Crandall syndrome (Pathology) - Hereditary deafness, pili torti (twisted hair) and hypogonadism due to deficiency of luteinizing and growth hormones

Marañon sign (Clinical Medicine) - Vasomotor response to stimulating the skin overlying the throat, commonly seen in Grave's disease.

Marine-Lenhart Syndrome (Pathology) - A toxic multinodular goiter associated with Grave's disease.

Möbius Sign (Clinical Medicine) - Impaired convergence of the eyes; seen in Grave's disease. Don't Confuse This With: Möbius Syndrome

Morgagni Syndrome (Pathology) - A variably polyglandular endocrine syndrome with the characteristic triad of internal frontal hyperostosis, obesity, virillism; typically occurs in women. Don't Confuse This With: Morgagni Disease, Glands, Globules

Nevo syndrome (Pathology) - Disorder characterized by excessive growth and gigantism during the first few years of life, along with mental developmental impairments. Don't Confuse This With: Soto's syndrome

Rabson-Medenhall Syndrome (Pathology) - Autosomal recessive syndrome characterized by insulin resistance due to insulin receptor mutation. Symptoms include genitomegaly and various developmental abnormalities of the bones, teeth, and skin (acanthosis nigricans).

Riedel Thyroiditis (Pathology) - This is a very rare disorder and the cause of this disease remains unknown. But on various studies, it has been demonstrated that antithyroid antibodies are present in the patient's blood, suggesting an autoimmune disorder as the culprit. This disorder affects mainly women and usually presents as a euthyroid condition. However, in a number of cases, it has been demonstrated that it can either present as a hypothyroid or hyperthyroid condition. The main characteristics of this condition include an extensive fibrosis of the thyroid gland and the surrounding neck structures. As a result, upon palpation of the thyroid, it has a very stone-like feel, which may be misdiagnosed as a malignancy. Don't Confuse This With: subacute lymphocytic thyroiditis, Hashimoto's thyroiditis, de Quervain thyroiditis

Rosenbach Signs (Clinical Medicine) - Three signs: closed eyelid tremor seen in hyperthyroidism; impaired ability to close eyelids on command during hysterical episode; and loss of abdominal skin reflex during bowel inflammation or hemiplegia. Don't Confuse This With: Rosenbach Test

Chapter 6: Environmental

Note: This chapter includes eponyms & buzzwords related to infection, nutrition, toxins, inanimate factors, and other environmental components.

Bancroft filariasis (Microbiology) - A filarial infection caused by Wucheria bancrofti. It often leads to extensive lymphedema of extremities and has also been given the name elephantitis.

Chvostek Sign (Clinical Medicine) - This a sign of tetany that can be seen in hypocalcemia and respiratory alkalosis. The sign is elicited by tapping the facial nerve at the angle of the jaw that will cause twitching of the ipsilateral facial muscle suggesting neuromuscular excitability.

Owl eye (Pathology) - Descriptive term for the Cowdry type A nuclear inclusions seen in cells infected with cytomegalovirus.

Rocky Mountain Spotted Fever (Pathology) - A parasitic infection causing a frontal and occipital headache, intense lumbar pain, continuous fever and a rash on extremities. Don't Confuse This With: Typhus

Trousseau sign (Clinical Medicine) Seen in hypocalcemia: to elicit the sign, a blood pressure cuff is placed around the arm and inflated to a pressure greater than the systolic pressure and held in place for 3 minutes, causing occlusion of the brachial artery. In the absence of blood flow, the patient's hypocalcemia will induce spasm of the muscles of the hand and forearm. The wrist and metacarpophalangeal joints flex, the DIP and PIP joints extend, and the fingers adduct.

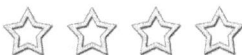

Addison Anemia (Pathology) - A disease caused by Vitamin B12 deficiency that results in megaloblastic anemia. It is also known as Pernicious anemia. Don't Confuse This With: Addison disease

Baghdad Boik (Microbiology) - Disease caused by a parasite-Leishmania that is transmitted through sand flies. This disease is also known as Leishmaniasis, orient boils, black fever, espundia, and sandfly disease.

Beriberi (Biochemistry) - Caused by Thiamine deficiency; Wernicke encephalopathy, emotional disturbances, weakness and pain in limbs, and irregular heart rate.

Caplan Disease / Syndrome (Pathology) - Occurs only in patients with both rheumatoid arthritis and pneumoconiosis related to mining dust (i.e.. coal, asbestos, silica) exposure.

Francis' Disease (Pathology) - Characterized by symptoms of sudden onset of chills, fever, weakness, headache, vomiting, and sweating which is caused by tularemia, a zoonotic disease.

Gambian trypanosomiasis (Microbiology) - Chronic infectious disease caused by Trypanosoma brucei gambiense in Africa with splenomegaly drowsiness, sleep sickness, psychosis, and often abnormalities in cerebellar and basal ganglia.

Korsakoff Syndrome / Psychosis (Pathology) - A brain disorder due to Vitamin B1 (thiamine) deficiency caused by severe malnutrition or chronic alcoholism. This disorder is also known as amnesic-confabulatory syndrome.

Leishman-Donovan Body (Microbiology) - Intracytoplasmic nonflagellated amastigotes of parasites such as Leishmania and Trypanosoma.

Mallory-Weiss Syndrome / Tear (Pathology) - Tears in the mucosa of the gastric-esophageal junction. These tears lead to bleeding and are caused by alcoholism and eating disorders that stretch the mucosa.

Wernicke Encephalopathy (Pathology) - This is a syndrome that includes short term memory loss amongst other symptoms. It is caused by lesions in the medial thalamic nuclei, mammillary bodies, periventricular and periaqueductal brainstem nuclei, and superior cerebellar vermis. These lesions are due to thiamine deficiency most often secondary to alcoholism.

Abercrombie Disease / Syndrome (Pathology) - A disease which includes amyloid degeneration including deposits of lardacein from tissues. It is seen in wasting diseases and indicates a problem in nutritive function. This is syndrome is also known as Bacony disease, cellulose disease, hyaloid disease, laraceous disease, or waxy disease.

Ackerman Tumor (Pathology) - This is a variant of squamous cell carcinoma. This cancer is seen in those who regularly use snuff or chewing tobacco. For this reason it is also known as Snuff dipper's cancer or Verrucous carcinoma. Don't Confuse This With: squamous cell carcinoma

Bang Disease (Pathology) - AKA Brucellosis. This is a zoonosis that is very contagious. It is caused by contact with infected animals or by ingestion of unsterilized meat or milk from animals that are in infected. It is also known as Undulant fever or Malta fever. Symptoms include fever, night sweats, malaise, anorexia, arthralgia, fatigue, weight loss, and depression, which can develop over days to weeks.

Bantu Siderosis (Pathology) - A iron overload disease that resembles hereditary hemochromatosis. It is seen in South African blacks that drank alcohol fermented in ungalvanized equipment.

Barlow Disease (aka. Moller Barlow, Infantile Scurvy) (Pathology) - A disease caused by a deficiency in Vitamin C.

Bitot spots (Pathology) - These spots are located in the conjunctiva and are a build up of debris from keratin. They are caused by Vitamin A deficiency and also associated with night blindness.

Burton Line (Pathology) - This is a sign of lead poisoning and is seen as blue discoloration of the border of the gingiva.

Casal Collar (Pathology) - A sign of niacin deficiency where a "collar-like" dermatitis is seen in the c3 and c4 dermatome region.

Chronic Mountain Sickness (Pathology) - A condition due to extended periods of stay at high altitude. It is characterized by hypoxemia and polycythemia.

Dum-Dum Fever (Microbiology) - See Baghdad boik.

Itai-Itai Disease (Pathology) - It is caused by cadmium toxicity. The disease is characterized by multiple fractures and a mixed scene of osteomalacia and osteoporosis. Renal damage is also seen.

Kashin-Bech Disease (Pathology) - A debilitating and permanent disease involving joint and growth cartilage. The cause remains unknown. However, some studies have proposed selenium deficiency, organic and inorganic salts in drinking water, and fungi to be possible causes.

Kerandel Sign (Clinical Medicine) - One of the initial signs of sleeping sickness (trypanosomiasis). There is delayed sensation of pain.

Kwashiorkor (Biochemistry) - Malnutrition due to insufficient protein nutrition in children; characterized by pot belly, hepatomegaly, depigmented skin, and commonly dermatitis.

Lash Casein Hydrolysate Serum Medium (Clinical Medicine) - A medium used to identify the presence of Trichomonas vaginalis. Don't Confuse This With: Lash Operation

Mad Hatter Syndrome (Pathology) - Chronic mercury poisoning causing gastrointestinal and CNS symptoms such as diarrhea, ataxia, and hyperreflexia.

Marasmus (Biochemistry) - Malnutrition due to energy deficiency; characterized by reduced body weight, normal height, and extensive tissue wasting.

Marburg Disease (Pathology) - (aka Marburg hemorrhagic fever) caused by Filovirus and characterized by similar symptoms seen in Ebola including multi-organ rashes and hemorrhages that are usually fatal.

Marchiafava-Bignami syndrome (Pathology) - A syndrome seen in severe chronic alcoholics whereby the malnourishment causes necrosis of the corpus collosum and white matter.

Mees' lines (Pathology) - These are discolored white lines appearing on the nails of the foot and hand. They are a sign of arsenic, thallium, or any other heavy metal poisoning.

Minamata Disease (Pathology) - A neurological condition caused by mercury poisoning. Symptoms include ataxia, numbness, general weakness, decreased visual field and damage to hearing and speech.

Monge disease (Pathology) - See Chronic Mountain sickness.

Onchocerciasis (Pathology) - The second leading cause of blindness in the world and is caused by Onchocerca volvulus. It is transmitted through the bite of the black fly and leads to worms being spread through the body. This is also known as River blindness.

Oroya fever (Microbiology) - Caused by gram negative bacilli: Bartonella bacilliformis; presents initially as a severe illness, associated with anemia. After, presentation with red-purple cutaneous nodular lesions.

Pastia Sign (Clinical Medicine) - Associated with scarlet fever, a transverse erythematous lines at the bend of the elbow, trunk and thighs that tends to persist after desquamation.

Pel-Ebstien Fever (Pathology) - A fever cycle that is associated with Hodgkin's disease whereby the fever lasts for a couple weeks and then the patient defervesce for the same period.

Russell Sign (Clinical Medicine) - These are scarred knuckles due to self-induced vomiting. The scarring occurs due to the knuckles being injured from the individual's teeth.

Schaumann Bodies (Pathology) - Are inclusion bodies found in the Langhans' giant cells, composed of proteins and calcium typically seen in granulomatous conditions such as sarcoidosis and berylliosis.

Vincent Angina (Pathology) - An infection of the gums due to an overpopulation of oral bacterial due to poor diet, smoking, and infection. It leads to inflammation, bleeding and necrosis of the gum tissues as well as fever and halitosis. This infection is also known as Acute necrotizing ulcerative gingivitis.

Whipple Triad (Clinical Medicine) - A triad of criteria that would suggest a patient's symptoms are related to hypoglycemia. The three stipulations posed are: Symptoms known to be caused by hypoglycemia; Low glucose measurement during symptoms; and Upon normal and raised glucose, there is a relief of symptoms.

Andrews' Disease (Pathology) - A rare sequel of a focal streptococcal or staphylococcus infection characterized by clusters of pustules on the palms of the hands that form a honeycomb pattern over time. Treatment is removal of the underlying infection.

Arneth Count/Index (Pathology) - This index describes the nucleus of a neutrophil. The index is used to determine different diseases such as B12/folate deficiency, infection or cancer.

Beurmann disease (Pathology) - A chronic disease caused by the fungus Sporothrix schencki. In one type, there is a lymphatic spread that involves the musculoskeletal system, gastrointestinal system, and nervous system. The pulmonary type is characterized by pneumonia.

Bilharzia (Pathology) - Parasitic disease caused by Schistosoma. This is also known as Schistosomiasis, bilharziosis, or Snail fever.

Carrion Disease (Pathology) - A disease caused by Bartonella species. This disease is also known as Bartonellosis, which is characterized by an initial life-threatening febrile phase, followed by an eruptive phase that produces hemangioma-like nodules in the skin and mucous membranes.

Chinese restaurant syndrome (Pathology) - Chest pain, facial pressure, and burning sensation from the reaction to MSG in food.

Chisso-Miamata disease (Pathology) - See Minamata disease.

Clapton line (Clinical Medicine) - Greenish discoloration of the gingiva in chronic copper poisoning.

Cruz' Disease/ Cruz Trypanosomiasis (Pathology) - See Chagas Disease.

Dagher Maneuver (Clinical Medicine) - A bimanual palpation maneuver to detect a foreign object that may be stuck in the pelvis.

Elsberg Syndrome (Pathology) - Neurologic impairment resulting in urinary retention that is associated with genital herpes.

Japanese Spotted Fever (Microbiology) - A febrile disease caused by Rickettsia japonica with rickettsial symptoms including acute high fever, headache and exanthema.

Lassa Fever (Pathology) - A severe, fatal form of fatal epidemic hemorrhagic fever caused by the Lassa virus; symptoms include sore throat, severe muscle ache, rash, hemorrhage, vomiting, diarrhea.

Lobo Disease (Pathology) - This is a fungal skin infection due to Lacazia loboi species, blastomycosis. Patient will present with keloidal nodular lesions on the face, ears or extremities. This is infection is also known as lobomycosis and lacaziosis.

Ludwig Angina (Pathology) - A life threatening cellulitis where there is an infection on the floor of the mouth in those with dental infections. A common cause includes most Actinomyces species. AKA Angina Ludovici.

Lutz-Splendore-Almeida Disease (Pathology) - It is also known as paracoccidioidomycosis.

Riggs' disease (Pathology) - A purulent and necrotic inflammation of the dental periosteum. This is also known as pyorrhea of a tooth socket and gingivitis expulsiva.

Schmorl Ferric-Ferricyanide Reduction Stain (Microbiology) - see Schmorl stain I.

Schmorl Stain I (Microbiology) - A stain used to test for tubercle bacillus.

Tietze Syndrome (Pathology) - This syndrome is characterized by a benign inflammation of the costal cartilages. The causes are not well known however stress and physical strain are associated with its symptoms of coughing, vomiting and chest injury.

Zieve syndrome (Pathology) - A relatively poorly understood disease. It has been associated with fatty liver/cirrhosis, severe upper abdominal and right upper quadrant pain, jaundice, hyperlipidemia, and hemolytic anemia. When excess alcohol ingestion is the main cause, the condition improves rapidly when alcohol consumption is stopped.

Addison-Biermer Anemia (Pathology) - See Addison's anemia.

Aldrich-Mees' Lines (Pathology) - See Mees' lines. Don't Confuse This With: Wiskott-Aldrich syndrome

Biermer anemia (Pathology) - See Addison's anemia.

Simmond Disease (Pathology) - See Sheehan Syndrome.

Virchow Syndrome (Pathology) - See Abercrombie's Disease/Syndrome. Don't Confuse This With: Virchow Node

CHAPTER 7: EYES & VISION

Notes: Eyes, Vision, and Eye-related signs are often among the most poorly understood topics by medical students. This chapter describes a topic that too-often gets nominal attention while studying for exams, which is exactly why a thorough study of this chapter can position you above your peers on exams and on the wards.

Argyll Robertson Pupil (Clinical Medicine) - A frequent sign of neurosyphilis; the patient presents with miosis and loss of both direct and consensual pupillary light reflexes; accommodation and convergence are retained. AKA Prostitute Pupil.

Haab Pupillary Reflex (Physiology) - Pupillary light reflex where there is contraction of the pupils due to a bright stimulus.

Kayser-Fleischer rings (Biochemistry) - Brown or green ring visible around the iris, due to copper deposition from Wilson's disease; copper deposition in Descemet membrane of cornea.

Lancaster Red-Green Test (Clinical Medicine) - Known commonly as red-green test, it is an ocular deviation test involving red and green filters over the eyes (red on right) to test for acquired strabismus and diplopia.

Lisch Nodule (Pathology) - Hamartomas on the iris; seen in type I neurofibromatosis patients.

Schlemm, Canal of (Anatomy) - Canal of the sclero-corneal junction, which receives the aqueous humor from the anterior chamber of the eye and returns it to blood circulation.

Fleischer Ring (Pathology) - Pigmented thin green or brown incomplete lines present in the corneal epithelium caused by the deposition of hemosiderin. Don't Confuse This With: Kayser-Fleischer Rings

Gifford Reflex (Physiology) - A reaction that occurs when the eyelids are forcefully held apart while an effort is made to close them, which results in constriction of both pupils.

Gillespie Syndrome (Pathology) - A condition characterized by the absence of the iris, mental retardation, and cerebellar ataxia, all present at birth, due to familial inheritance,

Meibomian Cyst (Pathology) - AKA Chalazian: usually occurs due to a blocked meibomian gland with resulting chronic granulomatous inflammation. Don't Confuse This With: Meibomian Glands (tarsal glands)

Reuss Color Chart (Clinical Medicine) - A chart specifically designed to in order to diagnose those with deficient color vision.

Snellen Chart (Clinical Medicine) - A test of visual acuity of distant vision using letters varying in size from the smallest on the bottom to the largest on top.

Vogt Syndrome (Pathology) - A form of corneal degeneration, due to inheritance, mainly affecting the Bowman membrane.

Wagner Syndrome (Genetics) - Variations in the peripheral fundus, pigmentation of the retina, circular membranes, and choroidal atrophy. Due to inheritance of a mutation in the gene encoding chondroitin sulfate proteoglycan-2

Wall-eyed bilateral internuclear ophthalmoplegia
(Pathology) - Lesions of both medial longitudinal fasciula (MLF) and a brainstem convergence centre; result is bilateral adduction weakness, exotropia.

Adie Pupil (Pathology) - The tonic pupil is the term used to denote a pupil with parasympathetic denervation that constricts poorly to light but reacts better to accommodation, such that the initially larger Adie pupil becomes smaller than its normal fellow and remains tonically constricted, redilating very slowly when exposed to dark. Don't Confuse This With: Argyll-Robertson Pupil

Behr Syndrome (Genetics) - An autosomal recessive disorder that causes bilateral optic atrophy with temporal field defects, nystagmus, ataxia, spasticity, and mental retardation.

Groenouw Corneal Dystrophy (Genetics) - A progressive autosomal dominant disorder with onset in early childhood; a granular type of corneal dystrophy characterized by punctuate opacities, corneal erosion, periodic photophobia, and foreign body sensation

Haenel Sign (Clinical Medicine) - One of the late stage symptoms seen in patients with tabes dorsalis as a result of neurosyphilis. No pain is felt when firm pressure is applied to the eye.

Harada Disease (Pathology) - An endemic disease of the far East. It mainly affects adults and is characterized by inflammation of the iris, ciliary body and choroid plexus. It is associated with meningoencephalitis.

Hering Law (Physiology) - States that corresponding agonist muscles of the eye are equally innervated while the antagonistic muscles are equally inhibited. Don't Confuse This With: Hering theory of color vision

Hutchinson Disease (Pathology) - A condition occurring with age in which the choroid degenerates with progressive and gradual loss of vision. Don't Confuse This With: Hutchinson Fracture, Pupil, Rule, Teeth

Hutchinson Pupil (Clinical Medicine) - On the side of the lesion, the pupil is fixed and dilated; may be due to an uncal herniation; oculomotor nerve is affected. Don't Confuse This With: Hutchinson Disease, Fracture, Rule, Teeth; Argyll-Robertson Pupil; Prostitute Pupil

Ishihara plates (Pathology) - plates used to test color vision, specifically red-green deficiencies, these plates contain a circle of dots of multiple colors with a number inside

Leber hereditary optic atrophy (Genetics) - A mitochondrially inherited disease that leads to progressive loss of central vision and blindness due to atrophy of the papillomacular bundle and the optic nerve.

Prostitute Pupil (Clinical Medicine) - Aka Argyll-Robertson pupils. Don't Confuse This With: Hutchinson Pupil

Rothmund Syndrome (Genetics) - An autosomal recessive inherited oculocutaneous disorder causing atrophy, pigmentation, and telangiectasia of the skin, congenital cataracts, congenital bone defects, and short stature

Small Disease (Pathology) - A disorder illustrated by visual impairment and modification to the retina which may include twisting vessels, exudative retinitis, neural deafness, muscle weakness, and mental retardation

Snellen Fraction (Clinical Medicine) - A ratio, determined by the use of the Snellen Chart, measuring the visual acuity of a person as compared to the standard or average ratio of a person with good eyesight

Stargardt Disease (Pathology) - The most frequently encountered juvenile hereditary macular dystrophy with macular degeneration leading to total blindness.

Tay Spot (Pathology) - In cases of Tay-Sachs' disease ,it is the appearance of the cherry-red spot on the retina.

Türk Syndrome (Pathology) - Fibrosis of the external rectus muscle due to congenital abnormalities of ocular and systemic origins. The patient is has limited abduction of the affected eye beyond mid-line.

Vogt Cornea (Pathology) - A form of senile corneal opacity that becomes present in old age

Waldeyer Gland (Histology) - Sweat glands associated with the eyelids

Wilbrand Knee (Pathology) - Possible artifact of retinal degeneration. Not a component of normal anatomy.

Wilder Sign (Clinical Medicine) - The presence of a twitch of the eye when moving from abducting to adducting; common in Grave's disease patients.

Zinn, zonule of (Anatomy) - Fibers from the inner surface of orbicularis ciliaris that run over the ciliary processes to the lens of the eye.

Arlt line (Clinical Medicine) - A linear scar present on the upper conjunctiva that is a classical sign of trachoma. Don't Confuse This With: Surgical scar, fibrosis

Brushfield spots (Clinical Medicine) - small white spots observed on the periphary of the iris in patients with Down's Syndrome.

Bumke Pupil (Physiology) - Transient dilation of the pupils, in response to anxiety or other psychic stimuli, and fails to respond to light and accommodation.

Chandler Syndrome (Pathology) - Is a rare eye disorder in which the single layer of cells lining the interior of the cornea proliferates, causing the drying up of the iris, corneal swelling, and glaucoma.

Cianca syndrome (Pathology) - Also known as infantile esotropia where one eye is medially rotated.

Cogan oculomotor apraxia (Pathology) - Inability to move the eyes in horizontal plane.

Cogan-Reese Syndrome (Pathology) - A condition in which the surface of the iris appears entangled or smudged, unilateral glaucoma in the eye which also has many peripheral anterior adhesions of the iris to the cornea, as well as the iris having multiple nodules and an ectopic Descemet membrane.

Collier sign (Clinical Medicine) - Midbrain lesion that causes a unilateral or bilateral lid retraction Don't Confuse This With: Collier's lung

Fleischer dystrophy I (Pathology) - Corneal dystrophy characterized by multiple brown lesions that spread towards the center of the orbit.

Foix syndrome II (Pathology) - Ocular disease resulting from intracranial aneurism and thrombosis of the cavernous sinus. Paralysis of the third, fourth, fifth, sixth, and ophthalmic branch of the fifth cranial nerve, associated with proptosis and edema of the eyelid.

Förster Choroiditis (Pathology) - Condition associated with syphilis causing inflammation involving the choroid and retinal vasculitis.

Foville-Willson syndrome (Pathology) - Impairment of abduction and mono-ocular nystagmus in the presence of disseminated sclerosis.

Fuchs coloboma (Pathology) - A congenital defect of the choroid at the inferior crescent on the edge of the optic disc. Don't Confuse This With: Myopia, Fuchs black spot, Fuchs Heterochromic Cyclitis

Goldmann-Favre Syndrome (Pathology) - An autosomal recessive inherited disorder characterized by progressive vitreoretinal degeneration, early onset of night blindness, and peripheral retinoschisis.

Haab Degeneration (Pathology) - An autosomal dominant form of localized extracellular amyloid deposition throughout the cornea. Presents with the 2nd or 3rd decade of life and doesn't begin to affect visual acuity for many years.

Hassall-Henle Bodies (Histology) - An outgrowth or enlargement at the margin of the cornea on the posterior surface of Descemet membrane; believed to be formed from collagen

Henle Warts (Pathology) - Small collection of hyaline in the periphery of the cornea. Found in those with degenerative disorders and chronic inflammation. Most likely associated with ageing.

Jaeger test types (Clinical Medicine) - Type of different sizes used for testing of acuity of near vision

Kearns-Sayer Syndrome (Pathology) - A mitochondrial disorder that generally manifests before the age of 20 years. It's a chronic progressive condition involving ptosis due to severe weakness of the muscles of the eyelids, retinal degeneration, short stature, hearing loss and cardiac conduction defects.

Krause Glands (Anatomy) - Accessory lacrimal glands.

Krunkenberg Spindle (Histology) - A vertical, spindle-shaped deposition of melanin pigmentation on the posterior surface of the deep layers of the cornea

Leber Congenital Amaurosis (Pathology) - A form of congenital blindness present at or shortly after birth; may be autosomal recessive in inheritance also characterized by searching nystagmus, enophthalmos, photophobia, and progressive retinal atrophy

Martegiani funnel (Anatomy) - The funnel-shaped dilation on the optic disc, from which the hyaloid canal begins.

Meibomian Glands (Anatomy) - Tarsal gland. Don't Confuse This With: Meibomian Cyst

Müller Fibers (Histology) - Supporting framework that forms the retina; consists of the fine fibers of the neuroglia cells. Don't Confuse This With: Müller Muscle

Müller Muscle (Histology) - The portion of the ciliary muscle that is innermost and consists of circular fibers Don't Confuse This With: Müller Fibers

Nettleship-Falls Albinism (Genetics) - A condition of ocular albinism that is sex-linked.

Pick Retinitis (Pathology) - A condition in which there is decreased visual acuity, reduced visual field with distortion of shapes, clouding of the retina, small hemorrhagic areas, distension of vessels, and peripapillary whitish grey macula. Don't Confuse This With: Pick Disease

Purkinje phenomenon (Physiology) - In the light-adapted eye, the region of maximal brightness is in the spectrum of yellow light; in the dark-adapted eye, the region of maximal brightness is in the spectrum of green light. Don't Confuse This With: Purkinje cells, fibers, figures

Ruysch Membrane (Histology) - Behind the retina this membrane is a very tight capillary network that composes a thin internal layer

Sakurai-Lisch Nodules (Genetics) - These nodules are seen on the iris with people that have type one neurofibromatosis

Sauvineau Ophthalmoplegia (Pathology) - A condition in which there is paralysis of the oculomotor muscles most closely associated with horizontal eye movements due to a lesion of the medial longitudinal fasciculus.

Schnyder Corneal Dystrophy (Pathology) - Is an autosomal dominant condition that presents with crystalline corneal degeneration. Some characteristics include grayish clouding of the cornea that stretches to the limbus and the presence of cholesterol deposits in the cornea.

Senior Syndrome (Pathology) - A congenital disorder characterized by a combination of nephronophthisis and retinitis pigmentosa.

Siegrist Spots (Pathology) - A string of pigmented areas lining white sclerosed choroidal vessels.

Tay Choroiditis (Pathology) - Slow progressive visual loss due to senile choroidal degeneration.

Thiel-Behnke dystrophy (Genetics) - Autosomal dominant condition characterized by slowly progressing anterior basement membrane damage of the cornea that leads to scarring, pain, and photophobia. This corneal dystrophy results in corneal opacities.

Trantas Dots (Pathology) - Small, pale, grayish-red or white-yellow chalky nodules of the conjunctiva around the limbus due to vernal keratoconjunctivitis.

Uhthoff Symptom (Clinical Medicine) - A condition occurring in those with multiple sclerosis during exercise where there is a temporary blurring of vision along with an increase in body temperature.

Usher Syndrome (Pathology) - Retinitis pigmentosa and sensorineural deafness due to autosomal recessive inheritance. It's considered the most common condition to affect both vision and hearing.

Valle Syndrome (Pathology) - Impairment of central vision due to recurring corneal reactions, however, peripheral retinal function remains intact.

Young-von Helmholtz Theory of Color Vision (Physiology) - A theory of color perception stating that there are three elements that are used to perceive color in the retina: red, blue, and green; Color perception is determined by the combined stimulation of the red, blue, and green elements.

Zöllner lines (Physiology) - Figures appearing as optic illusions (i.e. parallel lines appear diverging because of the placement of other lines around them). Don't Confuse This With: Zollinger-Ellison Syndrome

Agnew incision (Clinical Medicine) - In acute dacryocystitis (inflammation of the tear duct), an incision used to release pus and pressure from the lacrimal sac.

Coats' Disease (Pathology) - A developmental retinal vascular variance shown as yellow subretinal exudates and telangiectactic retinal vessels, conjunctiva, face, nail beds, and breasts. The progression of this disease slowly leads to atrophy, cataract, glaucoma, or retinal detachment. Don't Confuse This With: Small's Syndrome

Eales Disease (Pathology) - Sudden visual impairment due to peripheral retinal vessel hemorrhage with recurrent vitreous hemorrhages.

Elschnig spots (Pathology) - Yellow or red spots on the retinal pigment epithelium. These spots are seen in patients with chronic hypertensive retinopathy on fundoscopic examination. Their complaints include seeing "black spots" which may block their vision.

Forsius-Eriksson Albinism (Pathology) - Type 2 ocular albinism; A syndrome characterized by hypoplasia of macula lutea, nystagmus, myopia, fundusalbinismus, and color blindness.

Foster Kennedy Syndrome (Pathology) - A syndrome caused by a meningioma, causing unilateral ipsilateral atrophy of the optic nerve with contralateral papilledema and central scotoma.

Fuchs black spot (Pathology) - An area on the fundus oculi in the macular region where there is pigment proliferation due to degenerative myopia after macular hemorrhage. Don't Confuse This With: Fuchs coloboma, Fuchs Heterochromic Cyclitis

Fuchs Heterochromic Cyclitis (Pathology) - A congenital disorder characterized by heterochromia of the iris, inflammation of the iris and ciliary body, corneal degeneration, keratic precipitates, and often cataracts. Don't Confuse This With: Fuchs black spot, Fuchs coloboma

Haller circle (Anatomy) - Anastomoses of branches of short ciliary arteries on the sclera around the optic nerve's point of entry.

Hannover canal (Anatomy) - The potential space separating the ciliary zonule from the vitreous body.

Hering Test (Clinical Medicine) - A test involving binocular vision. Don't Confuse This With: Hering law

Hering theory of color vision (Physiology) - A theory that states there are three different sets of antagonistic color receptors: blue-yellow, red-green, and white-black. Don't Confuse This With: Hering law

Holmgren Test (Clinical Medicine) - A test for color blindness in which patient has to match colored skeins of yarn.

Horner-Trantas dots (Anatomy) - Imperceptible white cellular infiltrates in early keratoconjunctivitis. Don't Confuse This With: Horner's syndrome

Kuhnt spaces (Anatomy) - Shallow pits between the ciliary body and ciliary zonule that open into the posterior chamber of the eye.

Listing Law (Physiology) - Law stating that when the eye moves from one object of focus to another, it revolves around an axis perpendicular to a plane cutting both objects' line of vision.

Listing Reduced eye (Clinical Medicine) - A mathematical model of the eye for the purpose of simplifying retinal imagery calculations.

Meibomian Conjunctivitis (Pathology) - Frothy secretions and hyperplasia of the tarsal glands associated with chronic conjunctivitis

Möbius Syndrome (Pathology) - A neurological disorder which bilaterally causes facial paralysis usually due to an oculomotor disorder

Mooren Ulcer (Pathology) - Corneal thinning due to chronic inflammation in the periphery, which moves towards the center of the cornea. Pain is almost always associated with the onset of the ulcer.

Morgagni cataract (Pathology) - A hypermature cataract, with a hard nucleus and softened cortex, where the nucleus gravitates within the capsule

Nevin Syndrome (Pathology) - A condition characterized by external ophthalmoplegia, retinitis pigmentosa, and neurogenic amyotrophy. It can also be associated with heartblock.

Norrie Disease (Pathology) - A rare congenital blindness arising from bilateral masses of tissue arising from the retina or vitreous (malformations), opacity of the lens, and atrophy of the iris.

Parinaud Oculoglandular Syndrome (Pathology) - Unilateral conjunctivitis, retrotarsal conjunctival granulations, with preauricular adenopathy in tularemia, chancre, tuberculosis, cervical lymphadenitis, and fever. Don't Confuse This With: Parinaud Syndrome

Paton Syndrome (Pathology) - An early indication of tabes dorsalis shown as an irregular contraction of the pupil. It is also known as Gowers' Syndrome II.

Purkinje Figures (Clinical Medicine) - Shadows of the retinal vessels seen during transillumination of the sclera as dark lines on a reddish field. Don't Confuse This With: Purkinje Fibers

Robertson Syndrome (Pathology) - Aka Argyll-Robertson pupil.

Salzmann Dystrophy (Pathology) - Occurs in patients with existing corneal disease and presents with a characteristic nodular dystrophy of the cornea, which appears as an accumulation of bluish-white superficial nodules in the mid-peripheral region.

Siegrist Syndrome (Pathology) - A chorioretinopathy in exophthalmic hypertensive patients who show albuminuria due to trauma; characterized by granular pigmented spots present in the fundus.

CHAPTER 8: HEAD & NECK

Arnold-Chiari malformation (Pathology) - The downward displacement of the brainstem and cerebellum through the foramen magnum, sometimes causing hydrocephalus. Don't Confuse This With: Budd-Chiari Syndrome

Bell palsy (Pathology) - Facial muscle paralysis due to damage of facial cranial nerve (VII). Don't Confuse This With: Horner Syndrome

Corti, Organ of (Histology) - Collection of auditory receptor cells in the floor of cochlear duct.

Hangman Fracture (Pathology) - Cervical spine lesion through C2 pedicles.

Horner Syndrome (Pathology) - As a result of sympathetic palsy ipsilateral side of face exhibits ptosis, miosis, and anhydrosis. Don't Confuse This With: Horner-Trantas dots, Horner teeth; Bell palsy

Meniere disease (Pathology) - This disease affects the inner ear. Typical symptoms include hearing and balance disturbances, a feeling of pressure, and tinnitus. It is caused by increase of endolymph volume leading to increased inner ear pressure. Don't Confuse This With: Multiple Sclerosis, Schwannoma

Monro, Foramen of (Anatomy) - An opening between the third ventricle and each of the lateral ventricles. Don't Confuse This With: Foramina of Luschka and Magendie, Aqueduct of Sylvius

Purkinje cell (Histology) - Cells between molecular and granular layers of cerebellar cortex. Don't Confuse This With: Purkinje fibers, Purkinje figures

Rathke pouch (Anatomy) - Upgrowth of the ectodermal roof of the stomodeum that forms the adenohypophysis.

Sylvius, Aqueduct of (Anatomy) - A 2cm canal connecting the third to the fourth ventricle in the mesencephalon. AKA Cerebral aqueduct. If occluded, causes hydrocephalus.

Barany caloric test (Clinical Medicine) - Allows to test vestibular apparatus on each side separately by placing cold or hot water to elicit nystagmus.

Herring bodies (Histology) - Expansions at the end of unmyelinated nerve fiber in pars nervosa of pituitary gland.

Hunt syndrome (Pathology) - Viral infection of facial nerve (VII). Don't Confuse This With: Bell palsy

Hutchinson pupil (Pathology) - Dilated pupil as a result of trigeminal nerve palsy (III). Don't Confuse This With: Hutchinson fracture

Nelson syndrome (Pathology) - Pituitary adenoma resulting in hyperpigmentation, third nerve damage, and enlarging sella turcica.

Nissl bodies (Histology) - Collection of endoplasmic reticulum and ribosome granules in the nerve cell bodies and dendrites.

Pick disease (Pathology) - Cerebrodegenerative disorder, in which atrophy of frontal and temporal lobes result in dementia.

Rathke cleft cyst (Pathology) - Remnant of the Rathke pouch from the pituitary development.

Wernicke reaction (Pathology) - Damage of optic tract resulting in loss of pupillary constriction when the light is directed to the blind side of the retina only. Don't Confuse This With: Wernicke Area, Encephalopathy; Wernicke-Karsicoff Syndrome.

Beckwith-Wiedemann syndrome (Genetics) - A congenital overgrowth condition with a combination of macroglossia, macrosomia, ear pits, midline abdominal defects, nevus flammeus and neonatal hypoglycemia. The child is at an increased risk of childhood cancers such as Wilms tumor and hepatoblastoma.

Benedikt syndrome (Pathology) - Tremor associated with hemiplegia and oculomotor paralysis on the opposite side.

Bitot spot (Pathology) - Greasy white deposits on the conjunctiva of the eye due to vitamin A deficiency.

Bonnier syndrome (Pathology) - Lesion of Deiters nucleus causes ocular disturbances, deafness, nausea, thirst, anorexia, and vagus related symptoms.

Cockayne syndrome (Pathology) - Autosomal recessive defect to excision repair of DNA manifesting with dwarfism, mental retardation, optic atrophy, deafness, microcephaly, and sensitivity to sunlight.

Duret lesion (Pathology) - Hemorrhage in the fourth ventricle.

Epstein pearls (Pathology) - Small cysts on the palate of newborns.

Galen great cerebral vein (Anatomy) - Unpaired vein that starts in third ventricle and together with inferior sagittal sinus forms the straight sinus.

Griesinger sign (Clinical Medicine) - Edema around the mastoid process due to emissary vein thrombosis indicates thrombosis of the sigmoid sinus.

Hutchinson facies (Pathology) - Specific facial expression as a result of external ophthalmoplegia. Don't Confuse This With: Horner syndrome

Kiesselbach Plexus (Anatomy) - the network of capillaries located in Kiesselbach area of the nose.

Le Fort I fracture (Pathology) - A horizontal maxillary fracture. Don't Confuse This With: Le Fort II fracture, Le Fort III fracture

Le Fort II fracture (Pathology) - A pyramidal facial fracture. Don't Confuse This With: Le Fort I fracture, Le Fort III fracture

Le Fort III fracture (Pathology) - A transverse craniofacial disjunction fracture. Don't Confuse This With: Le Fort I fracture, Le Fort II fracture

Leigh disease (Pathology) - Autosomal recessive deficiency enzymes involved in energy metabolism causing seizures, spasticity, optic atrophy, and dementia in infants.

Lemon Sign (Clinical Medicine) - In ultrasound imaging, it is the scalloping of the frontal bone due to inward brain traction; common finding in Arnold-Chiari malformation.

Moll glands (Anatomy) - Apocrine glands in the eyelids, with secretary duct in the follicles of eyelashes.

Moon molars (Pathology) - Small dome-shaped first molar teeth occurring in congenital syphilis.

Quant sign (Clinical Medicine) - A T-shaped depression in the occipital bone seen in many patients with rickets and infants lying in bed.

Queckenstedt-Stookey test (Clinical Medicine) - Absence of increase of pressure in the cerebrospinal fluid when jugular vein is compressed in the block of subarachnoid channels.

Riddoch Phenomenon (Pathology) - Occipital lobe lesions may result in abnormal ability to observe a moving object in an area of the visual field blind to static objects. Although aware of movement, the person has difficulty with perception of what the moving objects are.

Robin Syndrome (Pathology) - Micrognathia that causes underdevelopment of the tongue and cleft palate, severe myopia, congenital glaucoma, and retinal detachment. Don't Confuse This With: Treacher Collins syndrome

Schwabach Test (Clinical Medicine) - Used in the assessment of hearing. Five tuning forks of different frequencies are used to assess the bone conduction of both ears.

Vernet syndrome (Pathology) - Posterior head injury results in paralysis of the motor part of the glossopharyngeal (IX), vagus (X), and accessory (XI) nerves.

Wharton Duct (Anatomy) - AKA submandibular duct.

Aicardi syndrome (Pathology) - X-link dominant disorder manifesting as agenesis of corpus callosum, chorioretinal abnormality, cleft lip and/or palate, and seizures.

Arnold reflex (Anatomy) - Stimulation of the sensory branches of vagus nerve in external auditory meatus causes a cough reflex.

Balint syndrome (Pathology) - Damage to superior temporal-occipital areas in both hemispheres results in difficulty with vision.

Bamberger sign (Clinical Medicine) - Sign of pericarditis with effusion when angle of the scapula is percussed for dullness that disappears with patient leaning forward.

Baumgarten glands (Anatomy) - Accessory lacrimal glands in the palpebral conjunctiva. AKA Henle glands. Don't Confuse This With: Bartholin Glands, Skene Glands

Bowman glands (Histology) - Serous glands in the olfactory region of the nasal cavity. Don't Confuse This With: Bowman capsule (kidney), Bowman membrane

Bowman membrane (Histology) - Cellular tissue layer under the epithelium of the cornea. Don't Confuse This With: Bowman capsule (kidney), gland, membrane.

Brunn membrane (Histology) - The epithelium of the olfactory region of the nose

Cajal, Nucleus of (Anatomy) - Group of nerves in the rostral end of the medial longitudinal fasciculus.

Canavan disease (Pathology) - Autosomal recessive inheritance, caused by mutation in the aspartoacylase A gene (ASPA) on chromosome 17p. Prevalent in Ashkenazi Jews. Manifests as megalencephaly, optic atrophy, blindness, psychomotor regression, hypotonia, spasticity, and increased urinary excretion of N-acetylaspartic acid.

Cestan-Chenais syndrome (Pathology) - Lesions of the brainstem affecting cranial nerves.

Conradi-Hünermann syndrome (Pathology) - Autosomal dominant disorder manifesting with skin keratinization and nervous system abnormalities.

Cooper-Rand artificial larynx (Pathology) - Electronic larynx.

Crooke granules (Histology) - Basophilic lumps in the anterior lobe of pituitary, associated with Cushion disease or administration of ACTH.

Dandy-Walker syndrome (Pathology) - Atresia of lateral foramina in 4th ventricle resulting in cerebellar hypoplasia and hydrocephalus.

Egyptian ophthalmia (Pathology) - Infection of the eye caused by Chlamydia trachomitis. Don't Confuse This With: trachoma

Fazio-Londe disease (Pathology) - Motor neuron degeneration causing bulbar palsy and affecting the brainstem.

Fothergill disease (Pathology) - Sensitive trigeminal nerve.

Foville syndrome (Pathology) - Midbrain lesions resulting in ipsilateral abducens paralysis and contralateral paralysis of extremities.

Fraser syndrome (Pathology) - Autosomal recessive disorder manifesting with cryptophthalmus with multiple anomalies, including middle and outer ear malformations, cleft palate, laryngeal deformity, displacement of umbilicus and nipples, digital malformations, separation of symphysis pubis, maldevelopment of kidneys, and masculinization of genitalia in females

Gardner-Wells tongs (Clinical Medicine) - Metal attachment for the skull, providing longitudinal traction in cases of cervical fracture

Goldenhar syndrome (Pathology) - Congenital anomalies manifesting as auricular appendices, unilateral posteriorly placed ear, unilateral microtia, atresia of external auditory meatus, and blind fistulae.

Gradenigo syndrome (Pathology) - Epidural abscess at the petrous pyramid causes compression of the abducens and trigeminal nerves.

Grunert spur (Pathology) - Outgrowth of the pupillary dilator muscle.

Guérin fracture (Pathology) - A maxillary fracture at the base above the apices of the teeth.

Horner Teeth (Anatomy) - A horizontal, hypoplastic groove on the incisor teeth. Don't Confuse This With: Horner's syndrome

Horton Test (Clinical Medicine) - Utilizing histamine to help investigate recurrent headaches.

Hyrtl loop (Anatomy) - In 1 in 10 people there is a communicating loop between the two hypoglossal nerves in the area of geniohyoid muscle. Don't Confuse This With: Hyrtl cell

KBG Syndrome (Pathology) - Is a rare condition characterized by facial dysmorphism, large than normal upper central incisors, costovertebral anomalies and developmental delay.

Kiesselbach area (Anatomy) - Located at the anterior portion of the nasal septum, containing a capillary plexus, commonly acting as the origin of epistaxis.

Kjer optic atrophy (Pathology) - Early vision loss transmitted as autosomal dominant disorder. Don't Confuse This With: Leber hereditary optic atrophy

Krause end bulb (Histology) - Cold sensitive nerve terminals in skin.

Lermoyez Syndrome (Pathology) - The incidence of increasing hearing loss and tinnitus before an episode of vertigo, and the return of such senses afterwards

Mendelsohn maneuver (Pathology) - Maintaining esophagus open by keeping the larynx at highest position during swallowing.

Meretoja syndrome (Pathology) - Multisystem disorder, including amyloidosis, corneal dystrophy, nerve palsies, and floppy ears.

Michel malformation (Pathology) - Hypoplasia of the petrous pyramid and aplasia of the inner ear.

Mikulicz Syndrome (Pathology) - Disorder characterized by inflamed salivary and lacrimal glands with xerostomia. Don't Confuse This With: Mumps, Sjögren syndrome

Moore lightning streaks (Pathology) - Shrinkage of vitreous humor causes photopsia as vertical flashes of light.

Morel ear (Pathology) - Large auricle with reduced grooves and thinned edges.

Newcastle Disease (Pathology) - Condition characterized by conjunctivitis, palpebral edema and inflammation caused by a single-stranded RNA avian virus.

Norrie disease (Pathology) - X-linked recessive disorder manifesting with bilateral masses arising from the retina and atrophy of the iris.

Nothnagel syndrome (Pathology) - Tumor of midbrain causing dizziness, staggering, and rolling gait.

Ohngren line (Clinical Medicine) - Imaginary line between the medial corner of the eye and the mandibular angle for classifying maxillary tumors.

Parinaud syndrome (Pathology) - Lesion of the superior colliculi causing paralysis of conjugate upward gaze. Don't Confuse This With: Parinaud Oculoglandular Syndrome

Raeder paratrigeminal syndrome (Pathology) - Similar to Horner syndrome but associated with trigeminal nerve (V) dysfunctions.

Russell Periodontal Index (Pathology) - Measuring bone loss around the teeth and gingival inflammation gives indication of the degree of periodontal disease present in the mouth.

Russell syndrome (Pathology) - Suprasellar lesions result in diminished growth in young children and loss of body fat.

Sanson images (Histology) - Reflections of light from cornea and anterior and/or posterior surfaces of lens.

Santorini, Vein of (Anatomy) - Bridging vein that passes through the parietal foramen, creating a connection between the superior sagittal sinus and the veins of the scalp. Don't Confuse This With: Santorini Fissures, Santorini Muscle, Santorini Duct

Scarpa Foramina (Anatomy) - Two boney canals that facilitate the passage of the nasopalatine nerves through the line of the intermaxillary suture. Don't Confuse This With: Scarpa's Fluid, Fascia, Ganglion, Membrane, Sheath, Staphyloma, Triangle

Scarpa Membrane (Anatomy) - This membrane covers the fenestra rotunda found in the tympanic cavity Don't Confuse This With: Scarpa's Fluid, Fascia, Foramina, Ganglion, Sheath, Staphyloma, Triangle

Schilder Disease (Pathology) - A fatal disease of the CNS that presents with adrenal atrophy and diffuse cerebral demyelination.

Schwartze sign (Clinical Medicine) - A pink tint that is observed behind the tympanic membrane. It can be associated with otosclerosis.

Simmonds disease (Pathology) - Similar to Sheehan syndrome.

Tapia syndrome (Pathology) - Paralysis of the larynx, palate, and tongue on one side.

Tornwaldt abscess (Pathology) - Chronic infection of the pharyngeal bursa causing nasopharyngeal discharge, occipital headache, and stiffness of posterior cervical muscles. Don't Confuse This With: Tornwaldt syndrome

Tornwaldt cyst (Pathology) - inflammation or obstruction of the pharyngeal bursa or an adenoid cleft with the formation of a cyst containing pus

Tornwaldt syndrome (Pathology) - see Tornwaldt abscess

Walther Ducts (Anatomy) - AKA minor sublingual ducts. Don't Confuse This With: Walther dilator

Water projection (Anatomy) - Radiographic view of the skull to emphasize the orbits and maxillary sinus.

Wyburn-Mason syndrome (Pathology) - Mentally retarded people develop arteriovenous malformation on the cerebral cortex, retinal arteriovenous angioma and facial nevus.

Anel Probe (Clinical Medicine) - A diagnostic probe used for nasal and lacrimal ducts.

Bednar apthae (Pathology) - Trauma induced infection of wounds. Often occurs from sucking the thumb or foreign objects against the hard palate in infants.

Bichat fissure (Anatomy) - The fissure that marks the hilus of cerebral hemisphere.

Bjerrum scotoma (Pathology) - Scotoma shaped like a comet's tail extending from the blind spot.

Caldwell-Luc operation (Pathology) - Procedure for opening into the maxillary antrum through the supradental fossa above the maxillary premolar teeth to remove tooth roots or abnormal tissue from the sinus.

Carabelli cusp (Anatomy) - A cusp located on the lingual surface of the mesiolingual cusp of upper first molars, varies in size from a pit to a large cusp.

Chamberlain line (Anatomy) - Imaginary line at base of skull running between the dorsal tip of the foramen magnum and the dorsal margin of the hard palate; normally lies above the tip of the odontoid process of this axis.

Claudius cells (Histology) - Columnar cells on the floor of the ductus cochlearis external to the organ of Corti.

Corti, Arch of (Anatomy) - The junction between the heads of Corti's inner and outer pillar cells, in the inner ear. Don't Confuse This With: Organ of Corti

Cupid bow (Anatomy) - Contour of the upper lip.

Dorello canal (Anatomy) - A bony canal sometimes found at the tip of the temporal bone. When present, it contains the inferior petrosal sinus and abducens nerve and connects to the cavernous sinus.

Ewart procedure (Pathology) - Tracheal tugging elicited by mechanical elevation of larynx.

Farabeuf triangle (Anatomy) - Area bounded by the hypoglossal nerve, the internal jugular vein, and facial veins where the bifurcation of the carotid artery can be seen.

Frankfort plane (Anatomy) - Imaginary plane passing through inferior orbital borders and superior margins of auditory meatus. Don't Confuse This With: Ohngren line

Granger line (Clinical Medicine) - Appearance of the optic chiasm groove on radiographs.

Henle glands (Anatomy) - See Baumgarten glands.

Hensen cell (Histology) - Supporting cells in the organ of Corti

Hopmann papilloma (Pathology) - Papillomatous growth in nasal mucous membrane.

Killian operation (Pathology) - Removal of anterior wall of frontal sinus and mucous membrane.

Lauth Canal (Anatomy) - Scleral venous sinus. Don't Confuse This With: Lauth violet

Little Area (Anatomy) - AKA Kiesselbach area.

Logan Bow (Clinical Medicine) - used post-surgery in repairing a cleft lip; arc-shaped wire attached to both cheeks to protect lip.

Lombard Reflex (Physiology) - Unconscious raising of voice intensity when speaking against a noisy background.

Martinotti cell (Histology) - Multipolar nerve cells distributed through the various layers of cerebral cortex with axons ascending towards the surface of the cortex.

Melnick-Needles osteodysplasty (Pathology) - Prominent forehead and small mandible as well as other issues with bones. Don't Confuse This With: Robin syndrome

Naffziger operation (Clinical Medicine) - Procedure whereby the lateral and superior orbital walls are removed to relieve severe exophthalmos.

Nagel test (Clinical Medicine) - A test for color vision using an instrument called the Nagel anomaloscope. Works by determining the amount of red and green that needs to be combined to match yellow.

Pulfrich phenomenon (Pathology) - Perception of an oscillating object moving in elliptical path when one eye is closed or does not see.

Reid base line (Clinical Medicine) - Line drawn in computed tomography from inferior margin of orbital through the auricle to the center of the occipital bone

Rieger Syndrome (Genetics) - A condition due to an autosomal dominant inheritance in which there is a malformation of the anterior chamber of the eye and the teeth, and iridocorneal mesenchymal dysgenesis.

Riga-Fede disease (Pathology) - Sublingual ulceration in infants. Don't Confuse This With: Bednar aphthae

Rivinus canal (Anatomy) - The major duct draining the anterior portion of the sublingual gland. Don't Confuse This With: Rivinus ducts

Rivinus ducts (Anatomy) - Ducts of sublingual salivary gland. Don't Confuse This With: Rivinus canal

Rosenthal, basal vein of (Anatomy) - Vein on the medial surface of temporal lobe that empties into the great cerebral vein.

Santorini, Fissures of (Anatomy) - Two vertical fissures present in the anterior portion of the ear canal, allowing for increased flexibility of the cartilaginous structures Don't Confuse This With: Santorini Duct, Muscle, Vein

Santorini, Muscle of (Anatomy) - Muscle fibers that run over the masseter muscle, applying lateral traction. Don't Confuse This With: Santorini Fissures, Duct, Vein

Scarpa Staphyloma (Anatomy) - A condition where the sclera bulges to the posterior of the eyeball due to degenerative changes seen in severe myopia. Don't Confuse This With: Scarpa's Fluid, Fascia, Foramina, Ganglion, Membrane, Sheath, Triangle

Tolosa-Hunt syndrome (Pathology) - Idiopathic granuloma causing cavernous sinus syndrome.

Wachendorf membrane (Anatomy) - Pupillary membrane.

Weiss Sign (Clinical Medicine) - See Chvostek sign

Wildermuth Ear (Anatomy) - An anatomical variant of the ear in which the anti-helix becomes dominant and the helix is backwards.

Willis cords (Anatomy) - Fibrous cords traversing the superior sagittal sinus. Don't Confuse This With: circle of Willis

CHAPTER 9: HEMATOLOGY

Auer Rods (Pathology) - Rod-like structures that stain red and are present in the cytoplasm of certain types of myeloid cells in cases of acute myeloid leukemia. They are most prominent in M3 Acute promyelocytic leukemia. Auer rods originate from the precursors to the granules in mature myeloid cells.

Basophilic stippling (Pathology) - Coarse or fine stippling with deep blue staining found in erythrocytes; sideroblastic anemia and lead poisoning.

Bence-Jones proteins (Pathology) - Immunoglobulin light chains that are rapidly excreted in the urine. Seen in multiple myeloma, renal failure, lytic bone disease, or malignant bone marrow cancer. May lead to secondary amyloidosis. Don't Confuse This With: Waldenstrom macroglobulinemia

Bohr effect (Physiology) - A fall in blood pH leading to a decreased affinity of hemoglobin for oxygen.

Burkitt Lymphoma (Pathology) - A highly aggressive childhood neoplasm of B-cells in lymph nodes caused by a MYC-IgH translocation (t:8,14) and involves the Epstein-Barr virus infection. Histology reveals a "starry sky" pattern of macrophages. Don't Confuse This With: Hodgkin Lymphoma

Coombs Direct antiglobulin test (Clinical Medicine) - Diagnostic test used to ascertain the presence of human antibodies or compliment on red blood cells; useful in detecting immunohemolytic anemia. Don't Confuse This With: Indirect Coombs test

Coombs Indirect antiglobulin test (Clinical Medicine) - Diagnostic test used primarily in pregnant women to detect unbound antibodies in plasma against red blood cells of known antigenicity. Don't Confuse This With: Direct Coombs test

Factor V Leiden (Biochemistry) - Mutation destroys the 2nd MnlI restriction site; hereditary thrombophilia; resistant to inactivation by protein C.

Heinz Bodies (Pathology) - Denatured hemoglobin that has precipitated on the red blood cell membrane and stains with supravital stain; found in G-6-PD deficiency; leads to "bite cells." Don't Confuse This With: Howell-Jolly bodies, basophilic stippling, Pappenheimer bodies

Hodgkin Lymphoma (Pathology) - Group of neoplasms that arise from a lymph node and spread to contiguous nodes. Characterized by the presence of Reed-Sternberg cells. Don't Confuse This With: Non-Hodgkin Lymphoma

Reed-Sternberg Cells (Pathology) - A large cell with a multilobulated nucleus and multiple nucleoli with a mirror image nucleus. They are characteristic of Hodgkin lymphoma and are surrounded by inflammatory cells.

Virchow Triad (Pathology) – A triad of factors contributing to thrombosis, including hypercoagulability, hemodynamic changes – typically stasis or intravascular turbulence, and endothelial injury. Don't Confuse This With: Virchow Node, Syndrome

von Willebrand Disease (Pathology) - An autosomal dominant disorder of spontaneous bleeding caused by absence or dysfunction of von Willebrand factors. Individuals with this disease have a defect in the coagulation pathway and are susceptible to spontaneous bleeding episodes. Don't Confuse This With: von Willebrand factor; Christmas disease, factor

von Willebrand factor (Biochemistry) - A large glycoprotein formed in Weibel-Palade bodies in endothelial cells that assists in the coagulation cascade by binding to clotting factors and facilitating the adhesion of platelets to damaged endothelium. Don't Confuse This With: von Willebrand Disease; Christmas disease, factor

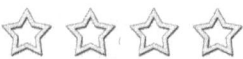

Christmas disease (Pathology) - Hemophilia B Don't Confuse This With: Christmas Factor, Hemophilia A

Christmas factor (Physiology) - Clotting factor IX Don't Confuse This With: Christmas disease, Hemophilia A

Faber Anemia (Pathology) - A form of anemia most commonly seen in middle aged women due to hemorrhagic disorders. Is due to lack of iron in the body causing koilonychias, pallor, premature graying of hair, and microcytic erythrocytes.

Hageman Factor (Biochemistry) - Factor XII Clotting factor.

Ham Test (Clinical Medicine) - The gold standard for diagnosis paroxysmal nocturnal hemoglobinuria. A positive test: lowering the pH will result in lysis of the patient's red blood cells.

Howell-Jolly bodies (Pathology) - Small dark nuclear remnants of DNA found in red blood cells with hereditary spherocytosis, asplenia, hemolytic anemia, and megaloblastic anemia Don't Confuse This With: Heinz bodies, basophilic stippling, Pappenheimer bodies

Huppert Syndrome (Pathology) - Multiple malignant tumors located in the bone marrow.

Pappenheimer Bodies (Pathology) - Cluster of excess iron that forms near red blood cell periphery indicating excess iron or sideroblastic anemia; stains with Prussian Blue stain. Don't Confuse This With: Howell-Jolly bodies, Heinz bodies, basophilic stippling

Weibel-Palade bodies (Physiology) - Cytoplasmic vesicles in endothelial cells that store von Willebrand factor. They play an important role in hemostasis and inflammation.

Cabot Ring (Pathology) - These are thin red violet rings found in erythrocytes. They are seen in individuals with erythropoetic disorders, lead poisoning, and megaloblastic anemia.

Ebola Virus (Microbiology) - Causative agent of Ebola hemorrhagic fever.

Hegglin Anomaly (Pathology) - An autosomal dominant, typically asymptomatic, leukocytic condition characterized by the presence of Dohle bodies in neutrophils and eosinophils, macrothrombocytopenia. Hemorrhagic tendencies may exist. Don't Confuse This With: Hegglin syndrome

Imerslund-Gräsbeck syndrome (Pathology) - Selective vitamin B12 malabsorption with proteinuria leading to juvenile megaloblastic anemia, autosomal recessive.

Kaznelson Syndrome (Pathology) - A congenital hypoplastic anemia associated with a microcytic, hypochromic blood smear.

Sezary Syndrome (Pathology) - Neoplastic CD4+ T-cells that home for the skin and are characterized by an exfoliative erythroderma and Sezary (tumor) cells in the peripheral blood. Don't Confuse This With: Mycosis Fungoides

Vaquez Disease (Pathology) - A chronic condition characterized by splenomegaly, redness or cyanosis of the skin, bone marrow hyperplasia, as well as an increase in blood volume.

Waldenstrom Macroglobulinemia (Pathology) - Condition of greatly increased blood viscosity due to large amounts of IgM in the serum. This is caused by lymphoplasmacytic lymphoma and manifests with visual impairment, neurological problems, bleeding, and cryoglobulinemia. Don't Confuse This With: Bence-Jones proteins; Multiple Myeloma

Waxy spleen (Pathology) - AKA amyloidosis of spleen. Don't Confuse This With: Waxy cast

Birbeck granules (Pathology) - Tubular structures with dilated ends (tennis racket appearance) that are found in the cytoplasm's of Langerhans cells in patients with Langerhans cell histiocytosis. Don't Confuse This With: Auer rods

Dacie Syndrome (Pathology) - Idiopathic massive splenomegaly Don't Confuse This With: Secondary splenomegaly

Donath-Landsteiner Antibodies (Pathology) - IgG antibodies that form in response to syphilis or viral infections that agglutinate in the cold.

Gaisbock syndrome (Pathology) - Also known as stress polycythemia that was characterized by normal RBC volume but decreased plasma volume.

Hemoglobin Barts (Pathology) - This hemoglobin has 4 gamma chains. It accumulated in RBCs and has a very high affinity to oxygen. This leads to severe decrease in oxygen allowance to the tissues. This is usually seen in hydrops fetalis.

Lancefield Classification (Microbiology) - Grouping system of hemolytic streptococci types by degree of group-specific carbohydrate precipitation

Letterer-Siwe Disease (Pathology) - Also known as acute disseminated Langerhans cell histiocytosis, is a form of this disease that is found in children less than 2 years of age Don't Confuse This With: Langerhans cell histiocytosis

Rabe-Salomon Syndrome (Pathology) - An autosomal recessive blood-clotting disorder that occurs from birth where there is bleeding from the umbilical cord which is due to the lack of fibrinogen synthesis.

Upshaw-Schulman Syndrome (Pathology) - A congenital bleeding disorder characterized by repeated episodes of thrombocytopenia and microangiopathic hemolytic anemia. This leads to jaundice, fever, systemic and renal hemorrhages, hematuria, confusion, paralysis and coma.

Werlhof Disease (Pathology) - previous term for idiopathic thrombocytopenic purpura

Alder syndrome (Genetics) - An autosomal recessive condition that stems from deficiencies in polysaccharide metabolism. Neutrophils show Alder bodies (dense azurophilic deposits) and is often associated with other mucopolysaccharide disorders such as Hurler's. Don't Confuse This With: Hurler Syndrome

Assmann Disease (Pathology) - Another name for myelofibrosis whereby the bone marrow undergoes fibrotic change resulting in an inability to produce new blood cells which then leads to myeloproliferative disorders.

Billroth, Cords of (Histology) - a.k.a. splenic cords, are found in the red pulp of the spleen in between the sinusoids, and consist of populations of monocytes and macrophages.

Di Guglielmo Disease (Pathology) - Is classified as an M6 subtype of AML involving massive numbers of nucleated red cells in the blood and bone marrow. Don't Confuse This With: Polycythemia

Diamond-Blackfan Syndrome (Pathology) - A congenital hypoplastic anemia due to a defect in the erythroid progenitor cells. Patients present with craniofacial abnormalities, neck anomalies, thumb abnormalities, genitourinary malformations and pre- and postnatal growth failure. Don't Confuse This With: Idiopathic aplastic anemia

Donath-Landsteiner Syndrome (Pathology) - An autoimmune syndrome caused by Donath-Landsteiner antibodies that results in abdominal and leg pain, hematuria, chills, fever, and pallor. Don't Confuse This With: Hemolytic anemia, pyelonephritis

Ehrlich Anemia (Pathology) - Anemia resulting from aplastic bone marrow. Don't Confuse This With: Aplastic anemia

Nasse Law (Pathology) - States that hemophilia occurs only in male progeny but is carried and transmitted through females, which are unaffected.

Neusser granule (Histology) - Small basophilic granules that form around the nucleus of a leukocyte.

Nikiforoff method (Clinical Medicine) - Method for fixing of blood films by immersion in alcohol, and/or ether.

CHAPTER 10: IMMUNE SYSTEM

Chediak-Higashi Syndrome (Pathology) - A rare, autosomal recessive disorder in which the patient suffers from recurrent infections, partial albinism, hepatosplenomegaly, an increased risk of lymphoreticular malignancy, and multiple neurologic abnormalities including but not limited to seizures, nystagmus and mental retardation. The defect involves the LYST gene.

Di George syndrome (Pathology) - A congenital immunodeficiency in which there are abnormalities of the face, congenital defects of the heart, hypoparathyroidism, cognitive, behavioral and psychiatric problems. This condition is a 22q11 deletion syndrome.

Ghon Complex (Microbiology) - Calcified lesion in hilar region and lymph nodes of the lungs, as a result from tuberculosis infection; this complex is formed in 2-3 weeks after initial infection.

Guillain-Barré syndrome (Pathology) - The most common type of acquired neuropathy originating as a delayed hypersensitivity autoimmune disease. It presents with progressive muscular weakness of the extremities, eventually leading to paralysis. The disease spreads proximally, and becomes life-threatening once the diaphragm is involved. Patients usually spontaneously recover.

Hansen Disease (Pathology) - AKA. Leprosy. A chronic disease affecting a host's immune cells. It is caused by Mycobacterium leprae. A diagnosis of leprosy should always be considered in any patient with skin lesions and/or enlarged nerve(s) accompanied by sensory loss.

Mantoux Test (Clinical Medicine) - It is also known as the tuberculin test. It checks for T cell response against Mycobacterium tuberculosis by injecting a purified protein derivative subcutaneously and observing a wheal and flare reaction on the skin in that area 48-72 hours later, indicating previous exposure to the antigen; example of type IV delayed hypersensitivity reaction.

Virchow Node (Clinical Medicine) - A palpable supraclavicular lymph node, especially on the left, that may signify a neoplasmic malignancy of the viscera. Don't Confuse This With: Virchow Triad

Bannwarth syndrome (Pathology) - Lymphocytic meningoradiculitis due to infection of Borrelia burgdorferi, which causes Lyme disease. Characterized by intense pain in the lumbar and cervical regions and radiating outwards. CSF abnormalities in the form of lymphocytic pleocytosis are also evident. Symptoms are facial paralysis, abducens palsy, anorexia, fatigue, headache, diplopia, paresthesia, and erythema migrans.

Behcet disease (Pathology) - A chronic condition caused by immune dysfunction. The immune system becomes overactive and unpredictable causing unknown and excessive inflammation, particularly small blood vessels, which lead to recurrent oral ulcers and genital, skin and eye lesions along with a positive pathergy test.

Bradley syndrome (Pathology) - Epidemic disease that usually occurs during the winter months and early spring at dawn. Symptoms include nausea, sudden and profuse vomiting, anorexia, constipation, pain, diarrhea, headache, and fever. It is believed that the syndrome has a viral etiology.

Bruton agammaglobulinemia (Genetics) - An X-linked recessive disease, where defective Bruton tyrosine kinase (Btk) protein leads to failure in B cell maturation in bone marrow.

CREST Syndrome (Pathology) - CREST is an acronym used to describe symptoms characteristic of scleroderma; C-Calcinosis (dermal calcium deposition), R-Reynaud phenomenon (vascular spasms due to temperature change), E-Esophageal dysfunction (including gastric reflux and dysphagia), S-Schlerodactyly, T-Teleangiectasias (dermal capillary dilation).

Felix' Reaction (aka. Weil-Felix) (Clinical Medicine) - Test used to diagnose typhus and other Rickettsial diseases. Determining the presence and type of the organism requires agglutination reaction based on common antigens.

Filatov disease (Pathology) - Epstein-Barr virus induced acute infection, presenting with fever, lymphadenopathy, and pharyngitis. It is also known as infectious mononucleosis. It can affect all age groups but is largely found in a younger population (20-25).

Herxheimer Reaction (Clinical Medicine) - A complication of antimicrobial treatment for Spirochetal bacteria that causes a systemic inflammatory reaction affecting dermal, mucous membranes and nervous system. Patient will present with fever, chills, headache, muscle pain and skin lesions. Don't Confuse This With: Steven Johnson Syndrome

Reiter Syndrome (Pathology) - Is a type of reactive arthritis with associated extraarticular manifestations in the eyes and urethra. Long term affects can cause cardiac manifestations including aortic regurgitation and pericarditis. Associated with Chlamydial infection.

Sjögren syndrome (Pathology) - A chronic autoimmune disease where immune cells attack and destroy exocrine glands that produce saliva and tears. It is characterized by xerostomia, pharyngolaryngitis, rhinitis, enlarged salivary glands, keratoconjunctivitis, dry mouth, dry nasal passages, dry skin, decreased sweating, and blocking of the Eustachian tubes, which may cause deafness. Don't Confuse This With: Mumps

Waldenström hyperglobulinemia (Pathology) - Autoimmune disease of the blood causing nonthrombocytopenic purpuric eruptions leading to the sedimentation of erythrocytes, increased gamma globulin levels in the serum, and thus mild anemia. Don't Confuse This With: Multiple Myeloma

Weinberg Reaction (Clinical Medicine) - A complement fixation procedure to test the presence of hydatid disease. Don't Confuse This With: Weil-Felix Reaction

Wiskott-Aldrich syndrome (Pathology) - X-linked recessive disease, characterized by eczema, immunodeficiency, and thrombocytopenia; involves mutation of WASP gene. Don't Confuse This With: Waldenstrom macroglobulinemia

Alder-Reilly bodies (Pathology) - Granular inclusions within polymorphonuclear leukocytes, which may be associated with Hunter and Hurler's syndrome and Morquio disease

Alibert disease II (Pathology) - An infection (may be dry or wet) caused by a sandfly carrying the Leishmania tropica parasite. The infection presents in the form of papules on the skin, which then becomes ulcerated and scabs.

Behçet syndrome (Pathology) - A recurrent disease of unknown etiology thought to be autoimmune in etiology, but also suspected to be caused by a microorganism. It is characterized by a triad of symptoms including uveitis, mouth ulcers and genital ulcers.

Bekhterev disease (Pathology) - A chronic autoimmune disease involving the spinal synovial joints, the margins of the intervertebral disks, and sacroiliac joints. It is characterized by arthritis, inflammation, and the eventual immobility of affected joints.

Boeck sarcoid (Pathology) - Benign systemic granulomatous usually affecting young adult females, and involving the lymph nodes, liver, spleen, lungs, skin, eyes, and salivary glands.

Brill disease (Pathology) - An infection caused by Rickettsia prowazekii that is transmitted by human lice or fleas. It is characterized by fever, transient rashes, and low blood pressure. Relapse occurs every 10-20 years. The disease can be seen in remote areas of Africa, Central and South America, and Middle and Western Asia.

Busse-Buschke disease (Pathology) - An acute or chronic infection of the CNS by Cryptococcus neoformans, which can cause a meningeal, pulmonary or disseminated mycosis.

de Almeida disease (Pathology) - It is a disease (blastomycosis) caused by the fungus Paracoccidioides (Blastomyces) brasiliensis. Ulcerations begin in the mouth and nostrils and spread downward to lungs, spleen, liver, GI tract, tonsils, and more. It commonly occurs in South American farmers.

Döhle bodies (Pathology) - Basophilic leukocyte inclusions in the periphery of neutrophils. They can be observed after Wissler's disease, May-Hegglin anomaly, Chediak-Higashi syndrome, burns, infections, trauma, and neoplastic diseases.

Ducrey disease (Pathology) - A sexually transmitted infection causing rupturing pustules at the genitalia due to infection by *Haemophilus ducreyi*.

Erb-Goldflam syndrome (Pathology) - An autoimmune disorder of unknown etiology where antibodies are made against acetylcholine receptors, thus causing ptosis, strabismus, complete ophthalmoplegia externa, weakness in the muscles of mastication, dysphagia, dysphonia, and muscular exhaustion.

Gardner-Diamond purpura (Pathology) - A chronic autoimmune syndrome that mostly affects women, characterized by recurrent painful ecchymoses of the body. Patient usually presents with tingling, itching, pain, and tenderness in their extremities. Some believe the disease is completely psychosomatic and there is no autoimmune component.

Haserick factor (Pathology) - Thermolabile antinuclear antibodies found in patients with Lupus erythematodes.

Hughes' syndrome (Pathology) - An autoimmune prothrombotic disease that can affect any vein or artery. It is possibly hereditary and caused by an anti-phospholipid antibody that is present individuals affected with this disease.

Hunter chancre (Pathology) - A papule on the penis, vulva, or cervix in primary syphilis.

Jurkat cells (Clinical Medicine) - T cells derived from Burkitt lymphoma, used in clinical research.

Kaposi-Irgang syndrome (Pathology) - A type of discoid lupus erythematosus where firm nodules can be seen under normal-looking skin. It frequently presents on the cheek. This autoimmune disease is two times more common in females.

Kikuchi's disease (Pathology) - Benign necrotizing lymphadenitis mainly affecting females. Characterized by non-cancerous enlargement of the lymph nodes caused by collections of proliferating histiocytes. The disease tends to resolve on its own within about 2-3 months.

Langhans Cells (Pathology) - Multinucleated giant cells present in granulomatous disease such as TB

Lederer-Brill disease (Pathology) - Autoimmune hemolytic anemia with extremely variable clinical features. Usually occurs in children after multiple infections.

Neisser-infection (Microbiology) - A sexually transmitted infection caused by the bacterium Neisseria gonorrhea. The disease is also known commonly as gonorrhea.

Pfeiffer meningitis (Microbiology) - Pfeiffer's bacillus induced meningitis.

Richter Syndrome (Pathology) - Presentation of pyrexia, weight loss, fatigue, lymphomegaly, and hepatosplenomegaly caused by the progression of chronic lymphocytic leukemia to large cell lymphoma.

Russell Bodies (Pathology) - Are dilated endoplasmic reticulum cisternae containing condensed immunoglobulins present in Waldenstöm macroglobulinemia.

Samter syndrome (Pathology) - Syndrome in asthmatic and allergic diseases, where bronchial asthma is found in addition to vasomotor rhinitis (with or without nasal polyps) and an intolerance to aspirin and similar medications.

Wagner-Unverricht syndrome (Pathology) - Autoimmune disease of the connective tissue and striated muscles, related to polymyositis, where skin turns purple or maroon. It is accompanied by fever, malaise, and an erythematous rash of the upper body. More common in females, children and the elderly.

Armstrong disease (Pathology) - Viral disease causing lymphocytic choriomeningitis.

Besredka vaccine (Clinical Medicine) - Vaccine used to prevent typhoid.

Cazenave disease I (Pathology) - Autoimmune disease of collagen that may be acute, but is more often chronic. It is also known as Luus de Cazenave or Lenoir's disease

Comby sign (Clinical Medicine) - Early sign of measles: white patches on the gums

Ducrey-Krefting bacillus (Microbiology) - The rod-shaped, gram-negative, bacteria causing chancroids or soft chancres of the Haemophilus genus. Don't Confuse This With: Ducrey disease, test

Ducrey test (Clinical Medicine) - Injection with Haemophilus ducreyi, subcutaneously, for diagnosis of chancroid. If hypersensitive, then it is indicative of a previous soft chancre occurrence. Don't Confuse This With: Ducrey disease; Ducrey-Krefting bacillus

Fanconi-Hegglin syndrome (Pathology) - Used to describe a nonspecific positive serology for syphilis in cases of viral pneumonias.

Fermi vaccine (Clinical Medicine) - A rabies vaccine.

Gänsslen disease (Pathology) - A type of constitutional leucopenia with an autosomal dominant basis. The disease can be asymptomatic, chronic with recurrent infections (especially of the gums,) or severe with generalized infections.

Gilbert syndrome 2 (Pathology) - Chronic pyemic colibacillosis resulting in entero-renal or entero-hepatic complications. This disease is caused by either foreign or native coli bacteria.

Glanzmann-Riniker alymphoplasia (Pathology) - Hereditary agammaglobulinemia with absence of the thymus, severe cytopenia, and susceptibility to infections by bacteria, fungus, and viruses. Antibodies will not form, and from early infancy there is a failure to thrive. Death usually occurs by the age of 2. Males are 3 times more susceptible to this condition, but inheritance can be autosomal recessive or X-linked.

Haffkine Vaccines (Clinical Medicine) - Anti-cholera serum and prophylactic plague vaccinations consisting of killed pathogen.

Hines-Bannick (Pathology) - Allergy characterized by excessive sweating followed by recurring episodes of hypothermia.

Kveim-Siltzbach Antigen (Pathology) - An extract found in the spleen, lymph node, or liver of patients with Boeck sarcoidosis that can be used for Kveim Test.

Kveim-Siltzbach granuloma (Pathology) - It is the formation of a granuloma as seen in sarcoidosis and occurs approximately 4 weeks after injection of Kveim antigen.

May-Hegglin anomaly (Genetics) - It is a rare genetic disorder causing thrombocytopenia due to abnormally large blood platelets. It is also associated with leukocyte abnormalities and leukocyte inclusion bodies.

Mollaret antigen (Microbiology) - Patients with cat-scratch disease produce this antigen from lymphatic matter.

Naegeli-de Quervain-Stalder test (Clinical Medicine) - Method used to demonstrate cell-combined allergic antibodies.

Neufeld Capsular Swelling (Microbiology) - Reaction in which encapsulated organisms may be visualized by the use of specific anticapsular antibodies. Don't Confuse This With: Quellung reaction, Neufeld reaction

Petzetakis' disease (Pathology) - An acute infection that occurs usually in young adults and children who have been bitten or scratched by a cat. Presents with regional lymphadenopathy and papules, chills, a slight fever, headache, anorexia, abdominal pain, and general malaise. Disease is self-limiting.

Petzetakis' disease (Pathology) - An acute infection that occurs usually in young adults and children who have been bitten or scratched by a cat. Presents with regional lymphadenopathy and papules, chills, a slight fever, headache, anorexia, abdominal pain, and general malaise. Disease is self-limiting.

Urbach-Königstein method (Clinical Medicine) - Diagnostic method for showing antibodies in allergies. Cutaneous allergen causes a local blister when a cantharidal dressing is placed on it.

Verneuil Disease (Pathology) - A chronic condition which results in multiple fistulous infected tracts due to an inflammatory response of the apocrine swear glands of the areolae, axilla, buttocks, groin, perineum, and umbilicus

Weil disease (Pathology) - Infection caused by Leptospira presents with jaundice, fever, oliguria, headache, myalgia, hemorrhaging. Disease is prevalent in males between their teenage years to adults. Vectors of transmission are rodents, skunks, dogs, foxes, and cattle. Characterized by jaundice, fever, oliguria, headache, myalgia, hemorrhaging, hepatosplenomegaly, and purpura.

Adamantiades-Behçet syndrome (Pathology) - See Behçet's syndrome.

Addison melanoderma (Pathology) - See Addison's disease.

Angelucci Syndrome (Pathology) - A non-bacterial conjunctivitis that usually occurs during the spring and is associated with hyperexcitability, tachycardia and vasomotor disturbances. Don't Confuse This With: bacterial conjunctivitis

Ardmore syndrome (Pathology) - Infectious disease probably caused by a viral infection that was first seen on a large scale at the Ardmore Air force base in Oklahoma.

Auer Phenomenon (Pathology) - After administration of Xylol, an allergic inflammation that is observed in sensitized rabbits. Don't Confuse This With: Auer rods

Bedsonia (Microbiology) - An infection caused by microorganisms of the genus Chlamydia that is responsible for lymphogranuloma venereum, trachoma, psittacosis.

Besnier-Boeck disease (Pathology) - See Boeck sarcoid.

Besnier-Tenneson syndrome (Pathology) - See Boeck sarcoid.

Boeck miliary lipoid (Pathology) - See Boeck sarcoid.

Boeck-Schaumann disease (Pathology) - See Boeck sarcoid.

Borovskii disease (Pathology) - See Alibert disease II.

Bruce septicemia (Pathology) - See Bang disease.

Cloquet, node of (Anatomy) - A deep lymph node located next to the femoral canal, sometimes mistaken for a femoral hernia when enlarged.

Cyprus fever (Pathology) - See Bang disease, Brucellosis.

Danaraj disease (Pathology) - See Takayasu arteritis.

Debre-Mollaret syndrome (Pathology) - See Petzetakis' disease.

Dreyfus-Dausset-Widal syndrome (Pathology) - See Lederer-Brill disease.

Durand-Nicolas-Favre disease (Pathology) - An obsolete term for a venereal disease found mostly in tropical and sub-tropical climates. The bacteria Chlamydia trachomatis characteristically infects the inguinal lymph gland with an exuding lesion. There are also non-venereal forms.

Dyke-Young syndrome (Pathology) - See Lederer-Brill disease.

E-rosette test (Clinical Medicine) - Method to identify human T-lymphocytes. Mixing blood lymphocytes with sheep erythrocytes causes rosettes of RBCs to form around human T-lymphocytes.

Endemic fever (Pathology) - See Brill's disease.

Fiedler disease (Pathology) - See Weil's disease.

Fiesinger-Leroy-Reiter disease (Pathology) - See Reiter's disease.

Foshay-Mollaret Cat-scratch fever syndrome (Pathology) - See Petzetakis' disease.

Frei bubo (Pathology) - See Durand-Nicolas-Favre disease.

Garin-Bujadoux syndrome (Pathology) - See Bannwarth syndrome.

Gilbert-Behçet syndrome (Pathology) - See Behçet's syndrome.

Goodall disease (Pathology) - See Bradley's syndrome.

Gougerot-Houwer-Sjögren syndrome (Pathology) - See Sjögren syndrome.

Hargraves' cells (Pathology) - Mature neutrophilic polymorphonuclear leukocytes that contain phagocytosed nuclei of other cells. These can be used diagnostically in acute disseminated lupus erythematosus.

Hayem-Widal-Loutit syndrome (Pathology) - See Lederer-Brill disease.

Heberden-Willan disease (Pathology) - See Henoch-Schönlein purpura.

Heller-Dohle messoaortitis (Pathology) - See Dohle-Heller syndrome.

Henoch disease (Pathology) - See Henoch-Schönlein purpura.

Hoppe-Goldflam syndrome (Pathology) - See Erb-Goldflam syndrome.

Hulusi-Behçet syndrome (Pathology) - See Behçet's syndrome.

Hutchinson-Boeck disease (Pathology) - See Boeck sarcoid.

Hutchinson-Boeck granulomatosis (Pathology) - See Boeck sarcoid.

Ito-Reenstierna test (Clinical Medicine) - See Ducrey test.

Jaccoud dissociated fever (Pathology) - Meningitis characterized by fever. In tuberculous meningitis, a slow pulse rate is also observed.

Königstein-Urbach reaction (Clinical Medicine) - See Urbach-Königstein method.

Kunkel syndrome (Pathology) - See Bearn-Kunkel-Slater syndrome.

Laënnec pearls (Pathology) - Term for round gelatinous masses in the sputum of asthmatic patients (obsolete).

Landouzy disease (Pathology) - See Weil's disease.

Larrey-Weil disease (Pathology) - See Weil's disease.

Leloir disease (Pathology) - See Cazenave disease I.

Loewenthal Reaction (Pathology) - Agglutination in patients with relapsing fever

Lupoide hepatitis (Pathology) - See Bearn-Kunkel-Slater syndrome.

Lupus de Cazenave (Pathology) - See Cazenave disease I.

Malpighian Bodies (Anatomy) - Splenic lymph follicles attached to smaller arteries. Don't Confuse This With: Malpighian pyramid, malpighian capsule, malpighian stratum

Malta fever (Pathology) - See Bang disease.

Marchiafava-Nazari-Micheli syndrome (Pathology) - See Strübing-Marchiafava-Micheli syndrome.

Marchiafava hemolytic anemia (Pathology) - See Strübing-Marchiafava-Micheli syndrome.

Marchiafava postpneumonic triad (Microbiology) - The concurrent occurrence of meningitis, endocardial ulcer, and septicemia in the lungs. Don't Confuse This With: Marchiafava hemolytic anemia

Martorell-Fabre syndrome (Pathology) - See Takayasu arteritis.

Mathieu disease (Pathology) - See Weil's disease.

Mediterranean fever (Pathology) - See Bang disease.

Moeller-Boeck sarcoid (Pathology) - See Boeck sarcoid.

Morbus Reiter (Pathology) - See Reiter's disease.

Mortimer disease (Pathology) - See Boeck sarcoid.

Mountain fever (Pathology) - See Bang disease.

Murine typhus (Pathology) - See Brill's disease.

Mylius-Schurman disease (Pathology) - See Boeck sarcoid.

Neapolitan fever (Pathology) - See Bang disease.

Nicolas-Durand-Favre disease (Pathology) - See Durand-Nicolas-Favre disease.

Pfeiffer disease (Pathology) - See Filatov disease.

Pierre Marie disease (Pathology) - See Bekhterev disease.

Raeder-Harbitz syndrome (Pathology) - See Takayasu arteritis.

Richet phenomenon (Pathology) - General anaphylaxis and sometimes fatal reaction occurring in a sensitized individual upon second injection of an antigen. It is also known as Theobald Smith's Phenomena.

Rotter Lymph Nodes (Anatomy) - Lymph nodes located in the space between the Pectoralis Major and Minor.

Say Syndrome (Pathology) - Characterized by a number of abnormalities including a chemotactic defect and a transient hypogammaglobulinaemia.

Schaumann syndrome (Pathology) - See Boeck sarcoid.

Searls' ulcer (Pathology) - See Bairnsdale ulcer.

Semple vaccine (Clinical Medicine) - Modified version of Pasteur's vaccine against rabies. It has severe side-effects and is not recommended by the World Health Organization.

Spencer winter vomiting (Pathology) - See Bradley's syndrome.

Sprunt disease (Pathology) - See Filatov disease. Strübing-Marchiafava-Micheli syndrome (Pathology) - A rare and chronic blood disorder characterized by hemolytic anemia, with attacks of nocturnal paroxysmal hemoglobinuria. The presence of dark urine is due to the degradation of erythrocytes

Theobald Smith phenomenon (Pathology) - See Richet's phenomenon.

Touraine aphthosis (Pathology) - See Behçet's syndrome.

Trisymptom Behçet (Pathology) - See Behçet's syndrome.

Turk lymphomatosis (Pathology) - See Filatov disease.

Unna-Ducrey bacillus (Microbiology) - See Ducrey-Krefting bacillus.

Vasiliev disease (Pathology) - See Weil's disease.

von Mikulicz-Gougerot-Sjögren syndrome (Pathology) - See Sjögren syndrome.

Waelsch urethritis (Pathology) - See Reiter's disease.

Wagner polymyositis (Pathology) - See Wagner-Unverricht syndrome.

Wassermann-positive pneumonia (Pathology) - See Fanconi-Hegglin syndrome.

Weil icterus (Pathology) - See Weil's disease.

Widal-Abrami-Lermoyez triad (Pathology) - See Samter syndrome.

Widal syndrome (Pathology) - See Samter syndrome.

Willis' disease II (Pathology) - Asthma. Don't Confuse This With: circle of Willis

CHAPTER 11: HEPATOBILIARY SYSTEM

Cori cycle (Biochemistry) - A metabolic pathway where lactate produced by anaerobic glycolysis from muscle circulates into the liver and is converted into pyruvate, supplying gluconeogenesis. Don't Confuse This With: Krebs Cycle

Kupffer cells (Anatomy) - Stellate-shaped cells lining sinusoids of the liver with phagocytic function; derived from monocytes.

Reye syndrome (Pathology) - Rare hepatoencephalopathy in children following an acute viral infection such as influenza or chicken pox, characterized by fatty liver, hypoglycemia, vomiting, agitation, lethargy, and possibly coma or death from edema and herniation of the brain; may be due to treatment of viral infection with aspirin.

Von Gierke disease (type I Glycogen storage) (Pathology) - Most common type of glycogen storage disease due to defect in glucose-6-phosphatase; absence of gluconeogenesis in liver, severe hypoglycemia, lactic acidosis, hyperlipidemia.

Andersen Disease (Pathology) - Glycogen storage disease IV, caused by transglucosidase deficiency.

Budd-Chiari Syndrome (Pathology) - Obstruction of hepatic vein by a space-occupying lesion causing liver cirrhosis and ascites.

Calot, Triangle of (Anatomy) - Occasional location of hepatic artery enclosed by inferior edge of liver, cystic duct and common hepatic duct.

Caput Medusa (Pathology) - This is the name given to the engorged veins radiating from the umbilicus on the surface of a distended abdomen. This is usually seen with portal hypertension as a result of cirrhosis.

Cori Disease (Pathology) - An autosomal recessive metabolic disorder classified as a glycogen storage disease III, characterized by debranching enzyme deficiency. Patients present with symptoms involving the liver and muscles.

Crigler-Najjar Syndrome (Pathology) - Disorder of unconjugated hyperbilirubinemia caused by one of either excessive bilirubin synthesis, defective bilirubin metabolism or abnormal bile. Patients are deficient in uridine diphosphate glycosyltransferase gene responsible for the conjugation of bilirubin. Don't Confuse This With: Dubin-Johnson Syndrome; Gilbert Disease

Dubin-Johnson Syndrome (Pathology) - An autosomal-recessive disease of conjugated hyperbilirubinemia caused by a defect in the bilirubin glucuronide transport protein Don't Confuse This With: Crigler-Najjar Syndrome; Gilbert Disease

Gilbert Disease (Pathology) - A hereditary disease causing unconjugated hyperbilirubinemia due to decreased glucuronosyltransferase (GT) in the liver Don't Confuse This With: Gilbert's sign; Crigler-Najjar Syndrome; Dubin-Johnson Syndrome

Hers Disease (Pathology) - Glycogen storage disease VI, due to phosphorylase deficiency

Ito Cells (Anatomy) - Hepatic fat-storing cells located in the space of Disse of the liver.

McArdle Disease (Pathology) - Glycogen storage disease V, caused by myophosphorylase deficiency

Meyenburg Complex (Pathology) - Bile duct hamartomas consisting of cystic dilation of the bile duct surrounded by fibrous stroma.

Rayer Disease (Pathology) - Cirrhosis, or scarring, of the bile ducts causing hypercholesterolemia, xanthomas and jaundice. Don't Confuse This With: Reye Disease

Rotor Syndrome (Pathology) - Autosomal recessive disorder of jaundice ad hyperbilirubinemia; resembles Dubin-Johnson Syndrome yet distinct by its lack of liver hyperpigmentation.

Schiff Biliary Cycle (Pathology) - Transport of bile salts from intestine to liver.

Tarui Disease (Pathology) - Glycogen storage disease VII, due to deficiency of phosphofructokinase.

Wilson disease (Pathology) - Autosomal-recessive disorder due to mutation in Wilson disease protein (ATP7B) gene; as a result, there is an accumulation of copper causing neuropsychiatric symptoms and liver disease.

Aagenaes Syndrome (Pathology) - Rare early onset genetic disorder involving underdeveloped lymph vessels that leads to intrahepatic cholestasis resulting in swollen legs and liver problems.

Addison-Gull Syndrome (Pathology) - A condition where scarring of the liver and bile ducts results in chronic jaundice, hepatosplenomegaly and yellow skin plaques due to abnormal lipid metabolism Don't Confuse This With: Addison Anemia, disease, melanoderma;

Bearn-Kunkel-Slater syndrome (Pathology) - An autoimmune chronic hepatitis seen in young women that is characterized by liver cirrhosis and extreme hypergammaglobulinemia with an increase in plasma cells. Onset is usually seen at puberty.

Bergmann-Eilbott test (Clinical Medicine) - Test of liver function by measuring bilirubin excretion levels.

Budd cirrhosis (Pathology) - Chronic hepatomegaly caused by intestinal intoxication. Don't Confuse This With: Budd's disease

Canal of Hering (Histology) - A ductule located between a bile canaliculus and an interlobular bile duct.

Caroli Disease (Pathology) - Hereditary liver disorder characterized by dilation of the large intrahepatic bile ducts. Also associated with liver fibrosis and renal cysts.

Fanconi-Bickel Syndrome (Pathology) - Glycogen storage disease type XI due to defect in GLUT2, accumulation of glycogen in liver and kidneys; glucose and glycogen are not utilized. This disorder of the liver involves renal Fanconi syndrome as well. Don't Confuse This With: Fanconi Disorder

Flint Syndrome (Pathology) - A hepatorenal syndrome developing in patients with severe liver disease (i.e.. alcoholic cirrhosis). Patients present with jaundice, dark urine and many other symptoms including delirium and confusion. Prognosis is poor.

Gilbert sign (Clinical Medicine) - A diagnostic test for liver cirrhosis whereby a positive test involves polyuria when fasting as opposed to post-prandially. Don't Confuse This With: Gilbert's disease

Glisson capsule (Anatomy) - The liver capsule (serosa) composed of connective tissue, sheathing the portal triad: hepatic artery, portal vein, bile duct. Don't Confuse This With: Glisson triad

Glisson triad (Anatomy) - The portal vein, hepatic artery and bile duct of the liver. Don't Confuse This With: Glissonian cirrhosis

Glissonian Cirrhosis (Pathology) - A form of perihepatitis that causes the liver capsule to thicken which leads to liver atrophy and deformity. Don't Confuse This With: Glissonitis

Heyd Syndrome (Pathology) - The onset of renal dysfunction caused exclusively by acute or chronic liver disease; symptoms include high serum creatinine and blood urea nitrogen, hyponatremia and hyperkalemia; all indicative of a loss in renal function.

Klatskin Tumor (Pathology) – AKA hilar cholangiocarcinoma: located proximally in the biliary tree, this tumor occurs at the convergence of the left and right hepatic bile ducts.

Laenecc Cirrhosis (Pathology) - Protruding nodules of parenchymal tissue on the liver surface, evident in alcoholic liver cirrhosis

Mallory Body (Clinical Medicine) - Prekeratin-containing inclusion bodies in liver cell cytoplasm staining eosinophically; characteristic of alcoholic liver disease, Wilson's disease, primary biliary cirrhosis or hepatocellular carcinoma Don't Confuse This With: Mammillary Body

Reynolds' Syndrome (Pathology) - A combined systemic sclerosis with primary biliary cirrhosis resulting in jaundice. Diagnostic testing includes the finding of high alkaline phosphatase levels.

Space of Disse (Histology) - A perisinusoidal space between sinusoids and hepatocytes of the liver housing Ito cells in plasma; liver diseases may lead to obstruction of this space

Zellweger Syndrome (Pathology) - Disorder of infancy whereby liver, brain and kidneys are deficient in peroxisomes. It is characterized by craniofacial dysmorphism and profound neurologic abnormalities.

Aguecheek Disease (Pathology) - Patients with liver disease who develop symptoms of dementia after eating a high protein diet due to an intolerance to the nitrogenous compounds found after the protein metabolism.

Baber Syndrome (Pathology) - A combined Fanconi syndrome and congenital liver cirrhosis which results in finger clubbing, skin hyperpigmentation and abdominal distension

Ballard Syndrome (Pathology) - Is a rare disease characterized by an enlarged liver and spleen, and weakened bone areas that have a high susceptibility to fracture.

Baumgarten's Syndrome (aka Cruveilhier-Baumgarten Syndrome) (Pathology) - Portal hypertension along with cirrhosis and splenomegaly leads to divergent circulation through the paraumbilical vein thus bypassing the liver.

Bean Syndrome (Pathology) - AKA Bean Dollar Bill Skin, Blue rubber bleb nevus: Is a disorder characterized by multiple subcutaneous and internal organ angiomas that can bleed and lead to anemia.

Byler Disease (Pathology) - Familial disorder of bile acid secretion that leads to cholestasis and progressive liver disease.

Cantlie Line (Anatomy) - Imaginary line bisecting the liver from the IVC to the left of the gall bladder fossa.

Frerichs' symptom (Clinical Medicine) - Symptom of Rokitansky disease, involving the presence of leucine and tyrosine in urine samples Don't Confuse This With: Frerichs' syndrome

Frerichs' syndrome (Pathology) - Renal dysfunction caused by acute or chronic cirrhosis of the liver. Don't Confuse This With: Frerichs' symptom

Glissonitis (Pathology) - Glisson capsule inflammation. Don't Confuse This With: Glissonian cirrhosis

Hanot Cirrhosis (Pathology) - Primary hypertrophic biliary cirrhosis caused by extra- or intrahepatic biliary duct obstruction, leading to liver fibrosis.

Touraine-Renault Syndrome (Pathology) - A condition that mainly manifests in middle aged males who are heavy drinkers or have liver dysfunction. It is characterized by painless lipomatous lesions of the trunk of the patient.

Mauriac Syndrome (Pathology) - Dwarfism, hepatosplenomegaly, and obesity seen in kids with uncontrolled diabetes.

Riedel Lobe (Anatomy) - Elongation of right liver lobe such that it points inferiorly and is palpable easily; considered to be either sessile accessory or a normal variant.

Westphal-Strumpell Disease (Pathology) - Aka. Wilson Disease

Chapter 12: Miscellaneous

Notes: This chapter includes eponyms & buzzwords pertaining to biochemistry, cellular biology, laboratory medicine, along with clinical instruments and tools.

Epstein-Barr virus (EBV) (Microbiology) - Herpes virus that is the causative agent in infectious mononucleosis and is implicated in Burkitt's lymphoma.

FISH (Biochemistry) - Fluorescent probes bind to specific genes of interest in chromosomes (Fluorescence in situ hybridization) Don't Confuse This With: ELISA; Northern, Southern, and Western Blot

Le Chatelier Law (Biochemistry) - For a system in equilibrium, changes in temperature and pressure cause adjustment in such a way that the system change is minimal.

Red Infarct (Pathology) – An ischemic infarct affecting tissues with dual blood supply, such as the lungs and intestines. The infracted area appears red due to reperfusion. Don't Confuse This With: White infarct

Southern blot (Biochemistry) - A molecular biology technique where DNA is electrophoresed on a gel and transferred to a filter; the DNA can be visualized on film through annealment of labeled DNA probe to electrophoresed DNA. Don't Confuse This With: FISH; Western Blot, Northern Blot

Western blot (Biochemistry) - A molecular biology technique where protein is electrophoresed on a gel and transferred to filter; protein can be visualized through the binding of labeled antibody. Don't Confuse This With: FISH; Northern Blot, Southern Blot

White Infarct (Pathology) – An ischemic infarct affecting solid organs, such as the heart, spleen, and kidneys. Reperfusion is minimal, and the infracted parenchyma appears white, rather than red. This is opposite to Red Infarctions seen in loose organs such as the lung and intestines. Don't Confuse This With: Red infarct

Ames' test (Clinical Medicine) - A test used to screen substances for potentially carcinogenic or mutagenic properties

Appian-Plutarch Syndrome (Pathology) - Another name for atropine overdose... remember some of the clinical signs "hot as a hare, blind as a bat, dry as a bone, red as a beet, and mad as a hatter."

Chocolate Agar (Microbiology) - A growth medium composed of lysed red blood cells, most commonly used for culturing of Haemophilus and Neisseria species. Don't Confuse This With: Thayer Martin agar, Blood Agar

Cooper ligament (Anatomy) – AKA suspensory ligament of Cooper: ligament that attaches to both the clavi-pectoral fascia and the dermis of breast tissue, providing support and shape for the breast.

Congo red (Pathology) - A stain used in microscopic preparations. Apple-green birefringence of this stain under polarized light is indicative of beta-pleated sheets of amyloid aggregates.

ELISA (Biochemistry) - Enzyme-linked immunosorbent assay; test for antigen-antibody reactivity. Don't Confuse This With: FISH

Eosin Methylene Blue Agar (Microbiology) - A growth medium for Gram-negative bacteria, allowing one to distinguish between lactose-fermenting and non lactose-fermenting bacteria. E. coli, specifically, gives off a distinct green hue when grown on this agar. Don't Confuse This With: Compare to Sorbitol MacConkey Agar or MacConkey agar

Giemsa Stain (Histology) - Methylene blue-eosin and methylene blue mixture used to stain for Negri bodies, spirochetes, and protozoans.

Golgi apparatus (Histology) - Cytosolic organ in eukaroyotes; membranous system of cisternae and vesicles situated between the nucleus and rough endoplasmic reticulum; assists in intracellular transportation of vesicle enveloped protein.

Hoyle Tellurite Agar (Microbiology) - Agar used for growth of Corynebacterium diphtheria. Don't Confuse This With: Thayer Martin Agar, Chocolate Agar, Blood Agar

Krebs cycle (Biochemistry) - Also known as the tricarboxylic acid cycle, occurring in the matrix of mitochondrion; integral in metabolic pathway for carbohydrate, fat, protein conversion. Don't Confuse This With: Cori Cycle

MacConkey Agar (Microbiology) - Growth medium used to differentiate lactose fermenting reddish colonies) from non-fermenting (colorless colonies) bacteria. Don't Confuse This With: Sorbitol MacConkey Agar

Mannitol Salt Agar (Microbiology) - A growth medium with high concentration of salt, conducive to selective growth of Staphylococci. Don't Confuse This With: Mannitol (osmotic diuretic)

Northern blot (Biochemistry) - A molecular biology technique similar to Southern blot, where sample RNA is electrophoresed instead of DNA.

Okazaki fragment (Genetics) - Short discontinuous segments of DNA synthesized away from the replication fork on the lagging strand during DNA replication.

Thayer Martin Agar (Microbiology) - Growth medium for Neisseria species on which Haemophilus species will not grow. Don't Confuse This With: Chocolate Agar

Weigert Stain for Elastin (Histology) - stain using fuschin, resorcin and ferric chloride, elastic ends up blue.

Weigert Stain for Fibrin (Histology) - a stain solution containing aniline-crystal violet and iodine-potassium iodide; fibrin ends up dark blue.

Blood Agar (Microbiology) - A growth medium for organisms that use hemolytic mechanisms for their nutrition. Don't Confuse This With: Chocolate Agar, Thayer Martin Agar

Hardy-Weinberg Law (Biochemistry) - Assumes (1) there is no mutation occurring in the allele (2) no preference or selection for any genotypes (3) mating is completely random (4) no net migration in or out of the population.

Hardy-Weinberg population genetics (Biochemistry) - Population equilibrium can predict disease prevalence: $p^2 + 2pq + q^2 = 1$; allele prevalence: $p + q = 1$; see Hardy-Weinberg Law.

Kahn Test (Clinical Medicine) - Quantitative test for syphilis. Not the most accurate test. Faster and simpler than Wassermann's test.

Leishman Stain (Clinical Medicine) - A type of stain used for blood smears that is composed of polychromed eosin-methylene blue.

Loffler Culture Medium (Clinical Medicine) - Used to isolate Loffler bacillus; contains beef blood serum, sheep serum, beef bouillon.

Sabouraud Agar (Microbiology) - Growth medium for fungi.

Sanger DNA sequencing (Biochemistry) - DNA sequencing with the use of dideoxynucleotides; ddNT terminate DNA polymerization at each base, generating various lengths of sequences of the original sample DNA; the various, terminated sequences are electrophoresed to find the original sequence.

Christian disease (Pathology) - Nodular fat necrosis.

Embden-Meyerhof pathway (Biochemistry) - The sequence of reactions in glycolysis in which glucose is converted to lactic acid.

Laroyenne Operation (Clinical Medicine) - Procedure involving puncturing the Pouch of Douglas to release pus in patients with pelvic suppuration.

Luft Potassium Permanganate fixative (Histology) - A fixative to preserve lipoprotein complexes in membranes and myelin.

Lugol Iodine Solution (Histology) - iodine-potassium iodide solution in histochemical staining; acts as an oxidizing agent.

Pfannenstiel incision (Clinical Medicine) – A horizontal surgical incision, with slight curvature, situated above the pubic symphysis and commonly used in C-sections.

Sachs-Georgi Reaction (Microbiology) - This is a diagnostic tool used in the identification of syphilis. It is a precipitation reaction that helps in identifying the lipoid antibodies that are characteristic to syphilis.

Schiff Base (biochemistry) - Condensation reaction between an aldehyde or a ketone and an aromatic amine.

Westguard Rules (Clinical Medicine) - A protocol of quality control that detects random and systematic error using 6 essential detector units

Altmann stain (Histology) - A stain used to visualize mitochondria.

Lauth violet (Biochemistry) - AKA thionine. Don't Confuse This With: Lauth Canal

Lister Method (Clinical Medicine) - Histological term for antiseptic surgery; originally performed under a cloud of dilute carbolic acid vapor.

Loffler Caustic stain (Histology) - See Loffler Stain.

Loffler Stain (Histology) - A stain for flagella.

Novy and MacNeal Blood Agar (Microbiology) - Nutrient agar suitable for the cultivation of some trypanosomes.

Passy-Muir valve (Clinical Medicine) - For patients who have undergone a tracheostomy, this is a speaking valve for them.

Randle Cycle (Biochemistry) - Oppositional relationship between the usage of glucose and free fatty acid in metabolism.

Walther dilator (Clinical Medicine) - Tapering instrument that dilates female urethra. Don't Confuse This With: Walther ducts

CHAPTER 13: MUSCULOSKELETAL

Ape Hand (Pathology) - Deformity of the thumb, limiting it to flexion and extension in the plane of the palm due to an inability to oppose or abduct the thumb, typically due to median nerve injury. Don't Confuse This With: Claw Hand

Battle Sign (Clinical Medicine) - Bruising immediately behind the ear (mastoid ecchymoses), indicative of a fracture of the base of the posterior skull with possible associated brain trauma. Don't Confuse This With: Raccoon Eyes

Bouchard Nodes (Clinical Medicine) - Abnormal boney or cartilagenous growths at the proximal interphalangeal joint, typically indicative of osteoarthritis. Don't Confuse This With: Heberden Nodes

Brittle Bone Disease (Pathology) - AKA Osteogenesis Imperfecta. Don't Confuse This With: Albers-Schonberg Disease; Marble Bone Disease

Brown Tumor (Pathology) - The hemorrhagic product of osteitis fibrosa cystica, a condition where normal bone is replaced by cysts and fibrous tissue as a result of hyperparathyroidism.

Claw Hand (Pathology) - A flexion deformity of the hand, resulting from damage to nerve roots C8 and T1. Don't Confuse This With: Ape Hand, Dupuytren Contracture

Duchenne muscular dystrophy (Pathology) - An X-linked form of muscular dystrophy, due to mutation of the dystrophin gene, rapidly progressing from onset in childhood. Most die in early adulthood. Don't Confuse This

With: Becker Muscular Dystrophy, Emery-Dreifuss Muscular Dystrophy

Ehlers-Danlos Syndrome (Pathology) - A genetic disorder (mainly autosomal dominant) of defective collagen synthesis. Characterized by hyperelasticity of the skin, hypermobility of the joints, easy bruising, and poor wound healing. Often associated with cardiovascular structural impairment. Don't Confuse This With: Marfan Syndrome, Osteogenesis Imperfecta

Heberden Nodes (Clinical Medicine) - Abnormal boney or cartilagenous growths at the distal interphalangeal joint, typically indicative of a degenerative bone disease (osteoarthritis). Don't Confuse This With: Bouchard's Nodes

Marfan Syndrome (Pathology) - An autosomal dominant disorder of connective tissue. Mutation in the FBN1 gene. Connective tissue throughout the body is affected but cardiovascular system is one of the systems with the most serious clinical manifestations. Fragmentation of the elastic fibers of the tunica media predisposes these patients to aneurysms and aortic dissection. The cardiac valves, especially the mitral valve, may become floppy and regurgitant. Patients typically present as tall a thin, with hyperextensile joints. Displacement of the lens of the eye is associated. Don't Confuse This With: Ehlers-Danlos Syndrome, Osteogenesis Imperfecta, Muscular Dystrophy

Paget Disease of bone (Pathology) - AKA osteitis deformans - A disease of osteoclasts, characterized by three distinct stages (osteolytic, mixed lytic and blastic, and osteosclerotic stages). Patients present with deformities, "chalk-stick" bones, fractures, and / or degenerative joint disease. Etiology is unknown but research implicates the paramyxovirus group of viruses as a causative agent. Don't Confuse This With: Paget's Disease (of Breast); Osteopetrosis, Osteomalacia / Rickets

Pott Disease (Pathology) - Tuberculous osteomyelitis affecting the spine, forming abscesses in multiple vertebrae and affecting surrounding soft tissue, including intervertebral discs.

Raccoon Eyes (Clinical Medicine) - Purplish discoloration around the eyes, indicative of fracture of the frontal skull base. Don't Confuse This With: Battle Sign

Scarpa Triangle (Anatomy) - An anatomical triangle consisting of the sartorius muscle, the anterior margin of the adductor longus muscle, and the inguinal ligament. Clinically important because it allows access to large vessels and nerves, and contains the potential space for femoral hernias. Also known as the Femoral Triangle. Don't Confuse This With: Scarpa's Fluid, Fascia, Foramina, Ganglion, Membrane, Sheath, Staphyloma

Unhappy Triad (Pathology) - Rupture of a triad of ligaments and meniscus at the knee joint: anterior cruciate ligament medial collateral ligament, and medial meniscus.

A Band (Histology) - An area of myofibril between two I bands that appears dark and has overlapping actin and myosin filaments. Don't Confuse This With: H Zone I Band, M Line, Z Disc, Z Line

Achilles Tendon (Anatomy) - AKA Calcaneal tendon.

Albers-Schonberg Disease (Pathology) - AKA Osteopetrosis. Don't Confuse This With: Brittle Bone Disease

Bamboo Spine (Pathology) - AKA Poker Spine - Rigid spine present in advanced cases of ankylosing spondylitis.

Becker muscular dystrophy (Pathology) - An X-linked recessive disease, characterized by muscular dystrophy due to defect in dystrophin protein; chronic progressive muscle weakness of legs and pelvis; onset in childhood; better prognosis than Duchenne muscular dystrophy. Don't Confuse This With: Duchenne Muscular Dystrophy, Emery-Dreifuss Muscular Dystrophy

Codman Triangle (Pathology) - A radiological indication of osteosarcoma, presenting as an elevated periosteal bone, forming a triangular shadow between periosteum and neoplastic cortex.

Colles Fracture (Pathology) - A transverse fracture of the distal radial metaphysis with dorsal displacement of the distal fragment, typically following a fall onto an outstretched hand. Don't Confuse This With: Smith Fracture

Crush syndrome (Pathology) - A syndrome caused by a serious and intense crushing injury to skeletal muscle. The syndrome includes shock and renal failure and is usually seen in victims of natural disasters. This is also known as traumatic rhabdomyolysis.

de Quervain tenosynovitis (Pathology) - Fibrosis and stenosis of the osseofibrous tunnel containing the adductor pollicis longus and extensor pollicis brevis.

Dupuytren Contracture (Pathology) - A shortening and hardening (contracture) of palmar fascia, typically forcing the ring and little fingers into a flexed position. Etiology is unknown, but is associated with liver. Don't Confuse This With: Ape Hand, Claw Hand

Emery-Dreifuss muscular dystrophy (Pathology) - A form of muscular dystrophy affecting both skeletal (contractures) and cardiac (impaired conduction, arrhythmias) muscle, caused by a mutation in nuclear envelope genes believed to be responsible for regulation of specific genes. Don't Confuse This With: Becker Muscular Dystrophy, Duchenne Muscular Dystrophy

Erb Palsy (Pathology) - AKA Erb-Duchenne Palsy, Brachial plexus paralysis - Paralysis of the arm induced by lesions to spinal roots C5-C7, usually during birth.

Gardner syndrome (Pathology) - An autosomal dominant mutation of the APC gene, resulting in familial polyposis colli, multiple osteomas, fibromas and fibrous dysplasia of the skull, and epidermal cysts. Don't Confuse This With: Osteoma, Osteoblastoma

Gorlin sign (Clinical Medicine) - Unusual extensibility in touching the tip of the nose with tongue; this may suggest Ehlers- Danlos syndrome.

Greenstick Fracture (Pathology) - An incomplete fracture of a long bone, with cortical disruption and bowing of the affected bone.

Guyon Canal (Anatomy) - Superficial osseofibrous canal between the flexor retinaculum and flexor carpi ulnaris, where the ulnar nerve and blood vessels pass Don't Confuse This With: Guyon Sign, Carpal Tunnel

H Zone (Histology) - The central portion of the A Band composed of thick filaments only, where actin and myosin fibers do not overlap. Don't Confuse This With: A Band, I Band, M Line, Z Disc, Z Line

I Band (Histology) - An area between to A Bands, containing the Z Disk (AKA Z Line, Z Band). Don't Confuse This With: A Band, H Line, M Line, Z Disc, Z Line

Jones Fracture (Pathology) - A fracture one inch distal to the proximal end of the fifth metatarsal, typically as a result of twisting inversion injury to the foot. Improperly managed Jones fractures typically do not heal well.

Lasègue Sign (Clinical Medicine) - It is also known as the Straight Leg Raise; used to diagnose sciatic nerve tension and lumbar intervertebral disc disorders

Ludwig Angle (Anatomy) - Sternal angle. Don't Confuse This With: Ludwig Ganglion

M Line (Histology) - The central portion of the H Zone, containing structural proteins within the thick filament portion of the sarcomere. Don't Confuse This With: A Band, H Zone, I Band, Z Disc, Z Line

Maffucci Syndrome (Pathology) - Enchondromatosis (Ollier Disease) associated with multiple soft tissue hemangiomas; thought to be associated with 100% chance of extra-skeletal neoplasms. Don't Confuse This With: Ollier Disease

Mallet Finger (Pathology) - AKA Baseball Finger - hyperflexion of the distal interphalangeal joint, resulting from avulsion injury to the long extensor tendon. Don't Confuse This With: Swan-Neck Deformity

Marble Bone Disease (Pathology) - AKA Osteopetrosis. Don't Confuse This With: Osteoporosis, Brittle Bone Disease, Vanishing Bone Disease

McArdle disease (type V Glycogen storage) (Pathology) - A glycogen storage disease due to myophosphorylase deficiency; weak muscles, cramps, myoglobinuria and rhabdomyolysis.

McMurray Test (Clinical Medicine) - A test to identify injury to the meniscal structures of the knee. A positive test presents as an audible click when the tibia is rotated in relation to the femur. Don't Confuse This With: Drawer Sign, Bulge Sign, Balloon Sign

Osgood-Schlatter Disease (Pathology) - AKA Osteochondrosis, Legg-Calve-Perthes Disease, Scheuermann Disease - A disease of the ossification centers of the bones of children, originally presenting with degeneration and necrosis, then with regeneration and recalcification.

Phalen Maneuver (Clinical Medicine) - Test for carpal tunnel syndrome performed by having patients hold both hands in acute flexion by pressing the backs of each hand together for 60 seconds or more. Don't Confuse This With: Tinel Test

Poupart ligament (Anatomy) - Also known as the inguinal ligament.

Saber Shin (Pathology) - A sign of tertiary syphilis, resulting from massive reactive periosteal bone deposition on the medial and anterior surfaces of the tibia.

Smith Fracture (Pathology) - AKA Reverse-Colles Fracture - an extra-articular transverse fracture of the distal radius with palmar dislocation of the distal fragment, typically as a result of a fall onto a flexed wrist. Don't Confuse This With: Colles Fracture

Tinel Test (Clinical Medicine) - Percussion of the median nerve at the distal portion folds of the wrist. Positive test indicates carpal tunnel syndrome Don't Confuse This With: Phalen Test

Trandelenburg Gait (Clinical Medicine) - Abnormal gait caused by a lesion of the superior gluteal nerve, typically resulting in weakness of the abductor muscles of the hip (gluteus medius and minimus). Don't Confuse This With: Magnetic Gait, Steppage Gait

Volkmann Canal (Histology) - A small canal, usually containing a vessel, connecting two Haversian Canals. Don't Confuse This With: Haversian Canal, Canaliculus, Glands, System; Volkmann Contracture

Volkmann Ischemic Contracture (Pathology) - AKA Volkmann Paralysis - Ischemic compartment syndrome of the forearm with flexion of the fingers and wrist, typically resulting from sudden occlusion or laceration of the brachial artery. Don't Confuse This With: Volkmann Canal

Weber Paradox (Physiology) - A muscle loaded beyond its ability to contract; it may elongate.

Z Line (Histology) - AKA Z Disc, Z Band - A darkly staining line in a myofibril, separating two sarcomeres. Don't Confuse This With: A Band, H Zone, I Band, M Line

Albright Hereditary Osteodystrophy (Pathology) - AKA Pseudohypoparathyroidism - End-organ resistance to parathyroid hormone, typically presenting with hypocalcemia, growth failure, and skeletal abnormalities.

Apley Scratch Test (Clinical Medicine) - A method for assessment of the range of motion at the shoulder joint, testing for capability of abduction with lateral rotation of one shoulder and adduction with medial rotation of the opposite shoulder.

Bankart Lesion (Pathology) - The most common reason of recurrent anterior dislocation at the glenohumeral joint, due to injury (avulsion) of the anterior capsule of the labrum.

Bardeleben bone (Anatomy) - AKA Os Trigonum - A small bone immediately posterior to the talus of the foot, commonly confused with a fracture of the talus.

Bennett Fracture (Pathology) - An intraarticular fracture of the first metacarpal that involves the first carpometacarpal joint. Don't Confuse This With: Rolando Fracture

Brodie Abscess (Pathology) - A form of cystic osteomyelitis, presenting as a small intraosseous abscess that typically involves the metaphyseal cortex and is walled off by dense granulation tissue and reactive bone.

Chance fracture (Pathology) - A flexion injury of the spine caused by violent forward flexion, resulting in transverse fracture of the posterior vertebrae and compression injury to the anterior portion of the vertebrae. Don't Confuse This With: Osteoporosis

Charley Horse (Pathology) - Cramping of the thigh muscle, typically resulting from a contusion, hematoma, or ischemia.

Cloquet hernia (Anatomy) - Femoral hernia behind the femoral vessels. Don't Confuse This With: Cloquet node

Ewing Sarcoma (Pathology) - A primary bone sarcoma of children and adolescents, belonging to the family of small round cell tumors, diagnosed by the characteristic t(11;22) translocation, which results in the dominant fusion oncogene: EWS-FLI1. This sarcoma is usually present in the long bones of lower limbs and does not present with osteoblastic activity. Don't Confuse This With: Osteosarcoma, Primary Neuroectodermal Tumor (PNET)

Fallen Arches (Pathology) - AKA Pes Planus - acquired flat feet.

Fanconi-Albertini-Zellweger syndrome (Pathology) - The syndrome includes osteoporosis with fractures, curving of long bones, growth retardation, heart defects, albuminuria, metabolic acidosis, and cerebrospinal fluid changes.

Felty Syndrome (Pathology) - Is characterized by rheumatoid arthritis, neutropenia and splenomegaly.

Finkelstein test (Clinical Medicine) - A test to diagnose de Quervain tenosynovitis (aka de Quervain disease): dorsal thumb pain elicited by thumb flexion and ulnar wrist deviation.

Fournier tibia (Pathology) - In congenital syphilis, thickening and anterior bowing of the tibia. Don't Confuse This With: Fournier's Gangrene, Fournier Sign

Gaenslen sign (Clinical Medicine) - Pain from hyperextension of hip upon flexion of opposite hip with fixed pelvis; torsion stress at sacroiliac and lumbosacral joints, testing for any abnormality with hip joints and femoral nerve.

Galeazzi Fracture (Pathology) - AKA Reverse Monteggia Fracture - Distal ulnar dislocation accompanying a radial fracture at the junction of the middle and distal portions of the radius, typically resulting from direct trauma from the dorsum or a fall onto an outstretched hand. Don't Confuse This With: Monteggia Fracture-Dislocation

Goalkeeper Thumb (Pathology) - See Skier's Thumb. Don't Confuse This With: Bennett's Fracture, Rolando Fracture

Gower Sign (Clinical Medicine) - Weakness of the proximal muscles of the lower limbs, with the patient requiring the use of his or her upper limbs to "walk" up his or her own body from a sitting or squatting position due to lower limb weakness. Suggestive of Duchenne muscular dystrophy.

Haversian Canal (Histology) - Small longitudinal canal present in long bone, containing blood vessels, nerves, connective tissue, and/or lymphatics. Don't Confuse This With: Haversian Canaliculus, System, Glands; Volkmann Canal

Haversian Canaliculus (Histology) - Tiny offshoots off of a Haversian canal, projecting into the lacunae of bone tissue. Don't Confuse This With: Haversian Canal, Glands, System; Volkmann Canal

Haversian System (Histology) - Concentric circular rings of lamellae and osteocytes located around a Haversian Canal, typically containing a central blood vessel. (see also osteon) Don't Confuse This With: Haversian Canal, Canaliculus, Glands; Volkmann Canal

Howship Lacunae (Histology) - Small irregular depressions on boney surfaces where osteoclasts accumulate and act to resorb bone. Don't Confuse This With: Haversian Canal, Canaliculus, System, Volkmann Canal

Jefferson Fracture (Pathology) - An burst fracture of the C1 vertebral ring, with fractures to both anterior and posterior arches, typically as a result of compression injury, often secondary to auto collisions

Kocher Maneuver (Clinical Medicine) - A rotation method consisting of three sequential movements (elbow traction, external rotation, adduction) to reduce a dislocated shoulder.

Lachman Test (Clinical Medicine) - aka Drawer Test (for Anterior Cruciate Ligament ONLY). Don't Confuse This With: Drawer Sign

Langenbeck Triangle (Anatomy) - Triangle shape formed by ASIS, greater trochanter and surgical neck of femur; common site of hip joint-related injuries

Lippman-Cobb Method (Clinical Medicine) - A procedure to measure the angle of scoliosis of the spine.

Little League Elbow (Pathology) - Medial epicondylitis. Don't Confuse This With: Little League Shoulder; Tennis Elbow

Lyme Arthritis (Pathology) - arthritis associated with Lyme disease.

Marie Disease (Pathology) - AKA Acromegaly. Don't Confuse This With: Marie Hypertrophy, Marie-Strumpell Arthritis

Marie-Strumpell Arthritis (Pathology) - AKA Ankylosing Spondylitis. Don't Confuse This With: Marie's Disease, Marie Hypertrophy

Monteggia Fracture-Dislocation (Pathology) - Proximal ulnar fracture with dislocation of the radial head. Don't Confuse This With: Galeazzi Fracture

Ollier Disease (Pathology) - AKA enchondromatosis - A syndrome of multiple enchondromas. Don't Confuse This With: Maffucci Syndrome

Onion Skin Appearance of Bone (Pathology) - Description of the bone seen on x-ray due to reactive bone formation in Ewing's Sarcoma.

Pitcher Elbow (Pathology) - Epicondylitis of the lateral epicondyle. Don't Confuse This With: Tennis Elbow

Plaster of Paris (Clinical Medicine) - The material, a white powder (Calcium sulfate hemihydrate), mixed with water to make a paste from which a cast can be made to immobilize a body part.

Pulled Elbow (Pathology) - Subluxation of the head of the radius with tear of the annular ligament, typically due to sudden jerking or lifting of a child's pronated arm.

Rolando Fracture (Pathology) - A comminuted intraarticular fracture of the first metatarsal involving the first carpometatarsal joint. Don't Confuse This With: Bennett's Fracture

Sever Disease (Pathology) - AKA Calcaneal Epiphysitis - A painful injury presenting in children as a disruption in the union of the cartilagenous layers of the epiphyseal plates of the calcaneus, typically resulting from athletic activity or excessive jumping.

Shin Splints (Pathology) - AKA Anterior Tibialis Strain - A mild form of anterior compartment syndrome, presenting as edema and pain, thought to be due to repetitive microfracture or muscular overuse.

Skier Thumb (Pathology) - AKA Goalkeeper's Thumb - Rupture of the ulnar collateral ligament of the first metacarpophalangeal joint, typically as a result of hyperextension of the joint. Don't Confuse This With: Bennett's Fracture, Rolando Fracture

Spring Ligament (Anatomy) - AKA Plantar calcaneonavicular ligament - important in maintaining the arch of the foot.

Steinert Myotonic Dystrophy (Pathology) - Progressive muscular wasting, myotonia, cataracts, mental decline, and hypogonadism due to familial inheritance.

Stoneman Disease (Pathology) - AKA Fibrodysplasia Ossificans Progressiva, Myositis Ossificans Progressiva - An idiopathic or inherited (autosomal dominant) systemic disorder of connective tissue in which bone replaces tendons, fasciae, and ligaments. Don't Confuse This With: Osteopetrosis, Paget's Disease

Student Elbow (Pathology) - Subcutaneous olecranon bursitis, resulting from repeated pressure and friction. Don't Confuse This With: Pitcher's Elbow, Tennis Elbow

Tennis Elbow (Pathology) - Epicondylitis of the medial epicondyle. Don't Confuse This With: Pitcher's Elbow, Student's Elbow

Ullrich Syndrome (Pathology) - An inherited muscular condition of childhood where, after birth, the child presents with contractures of the muscles of the neck and trunk, drooping of the head, kyphoscoliosis, and limpness of small joints while the large joints show contracture

von Recklinghausen disease (of Bone) (Pathology) - AKA generalized osteitis fibrosa cystica. Don't Confuse This With: von Recklinghausen's disease

Ward Triangle (Clinical Medicine) - Dark (radiolucent) area in x-ray plain films representing the trabecular pattern of the neck of the femur; indicative of osteoporosis.

Abadie sign of exophthalmic goiter (Clinical Medicine) - Spasm of levator palpebrae superioris muscle in Grave's disease. Don't Confuse This With: Abadie sign of tabes dorsalis

Abadie sign of tabes dorsalis (Clinical Medicine) - An absence of pain upon application of pressure or pinching of the calcaneal tendon, indicating Tabes Dorsalis. Don't Confuse This With: Abadie sign of exophthalmic goiter

Achard Syndrome (Genetics) - An autosomal dominant condition very similar to Marfan's Syndrome with the following differences: there is no abnormal height, eye or heart abnormalities, there is no subcutaneous fat abnormalities, the body is in proportion, and the skull is broad. Don't Confuse This With: Marfan Syndrome

Anatomical Snuffbox (Anatomy) - A superficial space found between the extensor pollicis longus and extensor pollicis brevis tendons upon concurrent contraction of their respective muscles. Tenderness may indicate fracture of the scaphoid bone.

Baker Cyst (Pathology) - Cystic swelling on the medial portion of the popliteal fossa, usually as an extrusion of synovial membrane from the knee joint cavity. May present with soreness and pain behind the knee.

Baller-Gerold Syndrome (Pathology) - Craniosynostosis with absence of the radius, due to an autosomal recessive disorder.

Barton Fracture (Pathology) - An intraarticular fracture of the radius with an oblique fracture line from the dorsum of

158

the radius to the radiocarpal joint, typically resulting from a fall onto an outstretched hand. Don't Confuse This With: Reverse Barton Fracture

Beals syndrome (Pathology) - An autosomal dominant dysplasia of bones, characterized by arachnodactyly with long thin bones, multiple contractures, kyphoscoliosis, and misshapen auricles.

Beevor sign (Clinical Medicine) - Neck flexion-induced movement of the navel superiorly, indicating weakness of the lower abdominal muscles

Blount disease (Pathology) - idiopathic growth disorder of the tibia (shin bone) in which the lower portion of the leg turns inward such that there is bowing of the legs.

Caffey Disease (Pathology) - AKA Infantile Cortical Hyperostosis - A disease of children characterized by areas of new bone growth underneath the periosteum, swellings and tenderness of the area, typically affecting the mandible, sometimes accompanied with a fever and irritability. Don't Confuse This With: Acromegaly

Caldwell-Moloy pelvic classification (Clinical Medicine) - A method of classifying the bony pelvic structure of a female, with possible classifications: android, anthropoid, gynecoid, and platypelloid, or a mixture of those four types.

Charcot Joint (Pathology) - Severe hypertrophic changes and sclerosis, due to ischemic necrosis, of the ankle and tarsal joints, typically secondary to diabetes. Characteristically presents with "6 D's" as follows: destruction, disorganization, dislocation, density (increased), distention (fluid), and debris

Charcot-Marie Tooth disease (Pathology) - Peroneal (fibular) muscular atrophy.

Chauffeur fracture (Pathology) - See Hutchinson fracture.

Chicken-Wire Pattern of Mineralization (of Bone) (Clinical Medicine) - A calcification of bony matrix, commonly near the knee, which is characteristic of Chondrobalstoma.

Chodzko reflex (Pathology) - Percussion of manubrium causes contractions of several muscles of shoulder girdle

Clado point (Anatomy) - Junction of the interspinous and right semilunar lines, at the lateral border of the rectus abdominis muscle. Clinically important in some cases of appendicitis, which present with tenderness and pressure at this point.

Cobb method (Clinical Medicine) - Determines the degree of curvature of the spine.

Codman tumor (Pathology) - Chondroblastoma of the proximal humerus. Don't Confuse This With: Codman triangle

Comolli sign (Clinical Medicine) - Triangular swelling found in scapula fractures.

Conradi disease (Pathology) - Hereditary chondrodysplasia with asymmetric calcification, dysplastic skeletal changes. Don't Confuse This With: Conradi-Hunermann syndrome

Crouzon Syndrome (Pathology) - AKA Branchial Arch Syndrome - A defect in the maturation of chondrocytes and osteoblasts due to a receptor (FGFR3) gene mutation, resulting in early fusion of cranial sutures and subsequent characteristic cranial deformities, with association to various ocular disorders.

Dunlop skin traction (Clinical Medicine) - A method of immobilizing the upper limb for orthopedic procedures like the correction of contractures or supracondylar fractures.

Dupuytren Fracture (Pathology) - Fibular Fracture near the tibiofibular synostosis.

Duverney Fracture (Pathology) - A stable ilial fracture inferior to the anterosuperior iliac spine. The pelvic ring remains intact, but with risk of hemorrhage.

Erlenmeyer Flask-Shaped Deformity (of long bones) (Clinical Medicine) - It is a deformity that occurs at the distal end of the femur and it is seen in Gaucher disease. It is an indication of osteopetrosis. Don't Confuse This With: Paget's Disease

Fairbank disease (Pathology) - Rare, idiopathic disorder mostly occurring in boys and is characterized by asymmetrical limb deformity due to overgrowth of cartilage, usually involving the lower extremities. Upon histological observation, the growth resembles osteochondroma. The clinical scenario involves stunted stature, painful joints and limited joint mobility. Don't Confuse This With: Fairbank-Keats syndrome

Fairbank-Keats syndrome (Pathology) - Rare, bone disease characterized by bone lesions that have a "hollowed out" radiographic appearance at the metaphases plates. The infant presents with failure to thrive, craniosynostosis, breakage of the vertebrae bones, and later on in life, dwarfism. Don't Confuse This With: Fairbank disease

Flatau syndrome (Pathology) - Autosomal recessive disorder characterized by bizarre movements of the trunk and neck, mostly manifests after physical activity.

Fong syndrome (Pathology) - AKA Nail-Patella syndrome - Absence or hypoplasia of the patella, dysplasia of nails, and bilateral iliac horns.

Forestier disease (Pathology) - Common condition in older men relating to the ossification of anterior spinal ligaments and tendons. Can manifest its self as ankylosing spondylitis.

Freiberg Infarction (Pathology) - A form of avascular necrosis, typically affecting the head of the second metatarsal unilaterally.

Gerdy Tubercle (Anatomy) - AKA Anterolateral Tibial Tubercle.

Gorham disease (Pathology) - AKA Vanishing Bone Disease - A rare congenital disorder characterized by endothelial proliferation of lymphatic channels that cause massive destruction and resorption of bone matrix.

Hajdu Syndrome (Pathology) - An autosomal dominant condition characterized by stunted stature, wormian bones and skeletal dysplasia. Joint laxity and bone fractures from minor trauma are key features.

Hench's syndrome (Pathology) - Sudden attacks of arthritis that may continue for a few hours or days and then disappear. Characterized by pain, no fever, redness, swelling, and an inability to move the affected joint.

Hill-Sachs Fracture (Pathology) - A fracture of the posteriolateral aspect of the humeral head following a strike of the humeral head into the inferior margin of the glenoid during humeral anterior dislocation at the joint.

Hollander Syndrome (Pathology) - A childhood disease of unknown etiology characterized by loss of subcutaneous fat in the face and trunk with either normal or excessive fat deposition in the pelvic region and lower limbs.

Homer-Wright Rosettes (Clinical Medicine) - Tumor cells arranged in a circle around a central fibrillary space, indicative of neural differentiation of neoplasms (i.e. Ewing sarcoma, medulloblastoma)

Housemaid Knee (Pathology) - AKA Prepatellar bursitis. Don't Confuse This With: Fong Syndrome

Hurler Cells (Pathology) - Characteristically seen in patients with Hurler's syndrome. The cells store heparan and dermatan sulfate.

Hutchinson fracture (Anatomy) - Radial styloid fracture.

Kast's Disease (Pathology) - Presence of multiple enchondromas and cavernous hemangiomas. Most cases are sporadic. Initial presentation is during childhood. Males are more frequently affected.

Kienböck's syndrome (Pathology) - A slowly progressive, degenerative disease of the lunate bone of the wrist. Young age of onset, usually following trauma. Patients presents with pain, stiffness, and limited range of wrist motion.

Kirmisson sign (Clinical Medicine) - Ecchymoses seen at the elbow in patients who fracture their humerus and the higher portion becomes displaced.

Klippel Deformity (Pathology) - Congenital abnormality whereby the scapula is abnormally high. Don't Confuse This With: klippel-trenaunay-weber syndrome

Kniest Syndrome (Pathology) - Congenital abnormality characterized by severe dwarfism and kyphoscoliosis. Patients present short trunk, prominent joints, flattened nose, delayed ambulation and cleft palate. Aka. Swiss Cheese Cartilage Dysplasia

Köhler's bone disease (Pathology) - An avascular necrosis affecting mainly the tarsal navicular bone as a result of constant compression cutting off blood supply and bone fragmentation. Onset is in early childhood.

Koslowski Syndrome (Pathology) - A form of dwarfism causing a skeletal abnormality whereby the trunk is extremely short. Also characterized by waddling gait, limited joint mobility and kyphoscoliosis. Don't Confuse This With: Kawasaki Disease

Kugelberg-Welander syndrome (Pathology) - A genetic, slowly progressive muscle weakness due to degeneration of ventral horn cells in the spinal cord. Don't Confuse This With: Duchenne muscular dystrophy

Kummell disease (Pathology) - Collapse of spinal vertebra post-trauma from even a minor injury. Occurs mainly in the middle aged and elderly.

Laband Syndrome (Pathology) - Autosomal dominant disease presenting as fibromatosis of the gums, hypoplasia of distal phalanges and dysplasia of nails; also causes joint hypermotility.

Lambrinudi Operation (Clinical Medicine) - A specific form of triple arthrodesis that prevents foot-drop.

Larrey Amputation (Clinical Medicine) - Amputation at the shoulder joint

Larson-Johanson Disease (Pathology) - Inflammation of lower pole of the patella caused by a developmental defect in ossification (osteochondroses), followed by traction forces that provide constant tension at the site of this immature bone.

Leri Sign (Clinical Medicine) - In hemiplegic patients, when wrist is passively flexed, flexion of unilateral elbow is impossible.

Lesshaft Triangle (Anatomy) - AKA Grynfeltt triangle; Superior lumbar triangle bordered by the quadratus lumborum muscle, the internal abdominal oblique muscle, and the transversalis fascia. Clinically, it is the site of lumbar hernias.

Lisfranc Injury (Pathology) - Tarsometatarsal joint injury, with or without an associated fracture. Don't Confuse This With: Lisfranc Amputation, Lisfranc Fracture-Dislocation

Maisonneuve Fracture (Pathology) - A disruption of the distal tibiofibular syndesmosis, the interosseous membrane, and a fracture of both the proximal fibula along with a medial maleolus fracture, typically a result of an eversion injury.

Marie Hypertrophy (Pathology) - AKA Hypertrophic Pulmonary Osteopathy - chronic periostitis-induced joint enlargement. Don't Confuse This With: Marie's Disease, Marie-Strumpell Arthritis

Meyenburg Disease (Pathology) - A rare inherited degeneration of cartilage resulting in arthritis and collapse of the ears, nose and tracheobronchial tree, which can lead to death by suffocation or infection. AKA Relapsing Polychondritis. Don't Confuse This With: Meyenburg Complex

Nelaton dislocation (Pathology) - Dislocation of the ankle, with the talus forced up between the separated tibia and fibula.

Panner disease (Pathology) - This is another name for osteochondrosis or avascular necrosis of the head of the humerus.

Popeye deformity (Pathology) - Rupture of the tendon of the long head of biceps resulting in the formation of a bulging mass (belly of the muscle) in the center of the anterior arm.

Reverse Barton Fracture (Pathology) - An intraarticular fracture of the distal of the radius with anterior dislocation of the carpals, typically as a result of direct trauma. Don't Confuse This With: Barton Fracture, Smith Fracture

Runner Knee (Pathology) - AKA Chondromalacia Patellae - soreness deep to the patella, resulting from quadriceps imbalance.

Schmorl Nodules (Anatomy) - Projection of the nucleus pulposus into the vertebra during kyphosis in adolescents.

Schober Sign (Clinical Medicine) - A test to check the flexibility of the lower back. It is mainly used when ankylosing spondylitis is suspected.

Sclerosing Osteomyelitis of Garre (Pathology) - A rare chronic disease, most commonly involving the mandible and resulting in extensive new bone formation with nonsuppurative periostitis that can obscure much of the underlying osseous structure.

Segond Fracture (Pathology) - A fracture of the lateral tibial plateau at the site of the attachment of the lateral capsular ligament, typically as a result of aversion injury at the knee. Don't Confuse This With: Unhappy Triad

Talma syndrome (Pathology) - Abnormal electrical excitability of muscles, resulting in prolonged contraction and decrease relaxation during rest. Usually develops in adults after trauma, intoxication, or acute infection.

Tennis Leg (Pathology) - Gastrocnemius strain resulting from a partial tear of the medial belly, typically at the musculotendinous junction. Don't Confuse This With: Tennis Elbow

Thomas Collar (Microbiology) - Splint used in fractures of the cervical spine due to tuberculosis infection. Don't Confuse This With: Thomas Sign

Thomas sign (Clinical Medicine) - Tuberculosis infection affecting the hip, resulting in formation of a compensatory curve of the spine upon extension of the damaged leg. Don't Confuse This With: Thomas Collar

Thomsen disease (Genetics) - An autosomal dominant condition manifests at infancy; characterized by spasms of proximal muscles of the limb, eyelids, and tongue;

aggravated by activity and provoked by cold. Associated with mutation in the Chloride channel 1 (CLCN1) gene.

Tillaux Fracture (Pathology) - Avulsion injury leading to fracture of the anterolateral portion of the distal tibia.

Van der Hoeve Syndrome (Pathology) - Stapedial fixation causing progressive hearing loss, starting in childhood; a subtype of osteogenesis imperfecta.

Volkmann Paralysis (Pathology) - See Volkmann Ischemic Contracture Don't Confuse This With: Volkmann Canal

Waldron Test (Clinical Medicine) - Creptiation at the patellofemoral articulation of the knee when passively flexing limb; seen in chondromalacia patellae.

Weber Fracture (Pathology) - Fibular fracture distal to the level of the tibiotalar joint, classified using the Weber Classification (Weber A-, B-, or C-type fractures)

Westphal sign (Clinical Medicine) - Absent or decreased patellar reflex

Wormian Bone (Anatomy) - Any tiny smooth bone, usually found at the serrated borders of cranial bone sutures.

Yellow Cartilage (Histology) - AKA elastic cartilage; a type of cartilage consisting of many elastic fibers giving it flexibility, found in the outer ear, larynx and epiglottis.

Aarskog-Scott Syndrome (Genetics) - An X-linked recessive disorder that results in physical abnormalities including: short stature, hand, foot, genital and face abnormalities. The afflicted have a round face with a broad nose and forehead, enlarged corneas, and a saddlebag scrotum. Health and developmental milestones are usually normal.

The mutation is in the FGDY1 gene on p11.21 of the X chromosome. Don't Confuse This With: Turner's Syndrome, Down's Syndrome

Allan-Herndon-Dudley syndrome (Pathology) - An X-linked recessive condition where the afflicted suffer from psychomotor retardation, hypotonia, a long, thin face, and hyporeflexia. Hypotonia presents at birth, with other symptoms following in months or years later. Don't Confuse This With: ALS

Apert syndrome (Pathology) - An autosomal dominant condition resulting in premature cranial development leading to craniofacial abnormalities accompanied by syndactyly or polydactyl. Don't Confuse This With: syndactyly, polydactyl

Ascher syndrome (Pathology) - A genetic disorder of children designated by the triad of: blepharochalasis, lip deformities, and non-toxic goiter.

Barlow Test (Clinical Medicine) - Test for subluxation or dislocation of the femoral head at the hip by adducting and extending the lower limb at the hip. This test is usually conducted on newborns to test for hip dysplasia.

Baseball Finger (Pathology) - See Mallet Finger.

Bennett hand tool test (Clinical Medicine) - A test of hand function, coordination, and speed used in occupational therapy. Don't Confuse This With: Bennett's Fracture

Boxer fracture (Pathology) - fracture of the metacarpal neck most classically seen in the 5th digit of the hand.

Bunnell Block (Clinical Medicine) - An orthotic device, typically used following surgery of flexor tendons of the hands to prevent flexion or joints proximal to those being exercised.

Bywaters' Syndrome (Pathology) - See Crush syndrome.

Cabot splint (Clinical Medicine) - A supportive metal splint worn on the posterior portion of the lower limb.

Camurati-Engelmann disease (Pathology) - AKA Diaphyseal Dysplasia - Thickening of the periosteal and medullary surfaces of long bones during childhood, sometimes with nerve tissue compression, typically presenting with weakness, pain, and wasting of the muscles of the lower limbs, all of which subside by early adulthood.

Carroll Quantitative Test of Upper Extremity Function (Clinical Medicine) - A six-part test using objects of different shapes and sizes designed to assess arm and hand movements which are needed for activities of daily life.

Chaput tubercle (Anatomy) - Attachment site for anterior tibiofibular ligament on the distal tibia. Don't Confuse This With: Charcot angina, disease, gait, joint, vertigo

Chopart amputation (Anatomy) - Amputation at the forefoot-midfoot junction.

Clark sign (Clinical Medicine) - Pain in patella indicative of chondromalacia patella.

Cleaves position (Clinical Medicine) - Radiographic technique visualizing shoulder joint without abduction.

Ely sign (Clinical Medicine) - Test for lateral thigh contracture. With patient in prone position, flexion of calf onto thigh causes retraction of gluteus maximus and abduction at hip.

Feil-Klippel syndrome (Pathology) - Congenital disease of unknown etiology having higher prevalence for females; characterized by reduced number of cervical vertebrae or fusion of vertebrae resulting in a short and wide neck with limited motion.

Greig Syndrome (Pathology) - A transcription factor gene (GL13) mutation, resulting in craniofacial abnormalities and syndactyly.

Hanhart syndrome (Pathology) - Several syndrome of variable inheritance, resulting in variable absence of digits or limbs, typically below the elbow or knee, along with high nose root, small eyelid fissures, and low-set ears.

Haversian Glands (Anatomy) - AKA Haver Glands - Extrasynovial fat deposits that may protect joint spaces. Don't Confuse This With: Haversian Canal, Canaliculus, System

Holt-Oram Syndrome (Genetics) - A transcription factor gene (TBX5) mutation, resulting in upper limb deformities and congenital skeletal abnormalities. Also known as heart-hand syndrome.

Jansen Metaphyseal Chondroplasia (Pathology) - A defect in the maturation of chondrocytes and osteoblasts due to a receptor (PTHrp) gene mutation, resulting in facial deformities, clinodactyly, and short bowed limbs.

Jarcho-Levin syndrome (Pathology) - A rare autosomal recessive disorder that is characterized by dwarfism, spine abnormalities (short thorax, rib defects), syndactyly. It is also known as spondylothoracic dysplasia. Death occurs as result of respiratory insufficiency.

Langer-Saldino Syndrome (Genetics) - AKA Achondrogenesis type II: autosomal dominant mutation in collagen type II gene, located on chromosome 12q.

Legg-Calve-Perthes Disease (Pathology) - See Osgood-Schlatter Disease

Lisfranc Amputation (Clinical Medicine) - Removing the foot at the tarsometatarsal joint while leaving the sole to function as a flap. Don't Confuse This With: Lisfranc Fracture-Dislocation, Lisfranc Injury

Lisfranc Fracture-Dislocation (Pathology) - A dorsal dislocation of the tarsometatarsal joints, often seen in parachute jumpers that severely plantarflex their feet upon landing. Don't Confuse This With: Lisfranc Amputation, Lisfranc Injury

Lisfranc, Scalene Tubercle of (Anatomy) - This is tubercle that is present on the first rib and is the site of attachment for the anterior scalene muscle. Don't Confuse This With: Lisfranc Amputation, Lisfranc Fracture-Dislocation, Lisfranc Injury

Little League Shoulder (Pathology) - Fracture of growth plate of humeral head, specifically in adolescents; caused by repetitive motions of pitching a ball. Don't Confuse This With: Little League Elbow

Luft Disease (Pathology) - Disease caused by uncoupled muscle phosphorylation; causes mitochondrial myopathy, excessive heat production, and hypermetabolism.

Macewen Triangle (Anatomy) - Useful landmark where the zygomatic arch meets the external acoustic meatus, which is used in mastoid operations. AKA suprameatal triangle. Don't Confuse This With: Macewen Sign

Malgaigne fracture of pelvis (Pathology) - Multiple pelvic fractures including the pubic rami and the ipsilateral ileum or sacrum.

McCune-Albright syndrome (Pathology) - AKA Albright Syndrome - presents with a combination of polyostotic fibrous dysplasia (due to GNAS1 mutation), hyperfunction of endocrine organ, and Café-au-lait spots Don't Confuse This With: Brown Tumor

McKusick Metahysial Dysplasia (Genetics) - aka (Cartilage-Hair Hypoplasia) autosomal recessive skeletal disease common in the Amish, with features of dwarfism, light colored hair, T cell defects, and metaphyseal dysplasia

Metenier Sign (Clinical Medicine) - Easy eversion of upper eyelids; indicative of Ehlers-Danlos syndrome. Don't Confuse This With: Meniere Disease, Menetrier Disease

Milkman Syndrome (Pathology) - Osteomalacia giving rise to many bilateral and symmetrical pseudofractures.

Morton Neuroma (Pathology) - A swollen and inflamed nerve at the ball of the foot, usually in the second intertarsal space. Don't Confuse This With: Morton Neuralgia, Morton Toe, Morton Syndrome

Morton Syndrome (Pathology) - Pain in the metatarsals due to congenitally shortened first metatarsal. Don't Confuse This With: Morton Neuralgia, Morton Neuroma, Morton Toe

Morton Toe (Anatomy) - First metatarsal is shortened in relation with second metatarsal; considered an anomaly with 10% population prevalence. Don't Confuse This With: Morton Neuralgia, Morton Neuroma, Morton Syndrome

Nance-Insley syndrome (Pathology) - Genetic disorder characterized by sensorineural deafness, large epiphysis, flattening of vertebral bodies, cleft palate, dwarfism and flat nasal bridge. Don't Confuse This With: Chondrodystrophy with sensoryneural deafness

Nance-Sweeney chondrodisplasia (Pathology) - See Nance-Insley syndrome. Don't Confuse This With: Chondrodystrophy with sensoryneural deafness

Oppenheim Disease (Pathology) - AKA Amyotonia Congenita: congenital pseudoparalysis that in infants is seen as lack of muscle tone where there is normally spinal nerve innervation. Don't Confuse This With: Oppenheim Reflex

Otto Disease (Pathology) - when the acetabulum bulges into the pelvis, associated with rheumatoid arthritis of the hip joint.

Patrick sign (Clinical Medicine) - Pain in the hip upon external rotation, can radiate to the back.

Pelligrini-Steida Disease (Pathology) - Ossification of the medial collateral ligament (MCL) as a result of chronic trauma to the MCL, typically as a result of avulsion injury at the origin of the MCL at the medial femoral condyle.

Pouteau Fracture (Pathology) - See Colles Fracture Don't Confuse This With: Smith Fracture

Prussak space (Anatomy) - Small middle ear recess that is bordered by the Shrapnell's membrane, the lateral malleal ligament, and the malleus.

Roberts' Pseudothalidomide Syndrome (Pathology) - Autosomal recessive disorder presenting with low birth weight, absence of long bones in arms and legs, severe mental retardation, ocular abnormalities, and cleft lip and palate; limited life expectancy. Don't Confuse This With: Roger's Disease

Russell-Silver Syndrome (Pathology) - Type of dwarfism associated with low birth weight, bilateral asymmetry, delayed anterior fontanel closure, and carp mouth.

Scaglietti-Dagnini syndrome (Pathology) - Acromegaly that causes hypertrophy of the clavicle, vertebral bodies, and the IV discs. A secondary condition may result known as cervical spondylosis.

Schanz' Disease (Pathology) - Inflammation of the Achilles tendon secondary to trauma.

Scheuermann Disease (Pathology) - See Osgood-Schlatter Disease.

Schlatter Disease (Pathology) - see Osgood-Schlatter disease.

Schmid Metaphyseal Chondrodysplasia (Pathology) - A collagen type 10 mutation, resulting in bowing of lower limbs, mildly-shorter stature, coxa vara, metaphyseal flaring.

Schmorl disease (Pathology) - Herniation of the nucleus pulposus.

Schmorl Stain II (Pathology) - a stain used to detect compact bone.

Schober manipulation (Pathology) - see Schober sign.

Schober Symptom (Pathology) - see Schober sign.

Stickler Syndrome (Pathology) - A collagen type 2 mutation resulting in premature osteoarthritis, flattened face, hearing loss, retinal detachment, and, commonly, myopia.

Waardenburg Syndrome (Pathology) - A transcription factor gene (PAX-3) mutation, resulting in craniofacial abnormalities, defective hearing, and abnormal pigmentation.

Weaver Bottom (Clinical Medicine) - Tenderness of the superficial ischiogluteal bursa, indicating bursitis.

Weber Classification (Clinical Medicine) - Classification used to determine the level of damage to the tibiofibular ligament, based on the severity of fibular fracture along with associated medial maleolus fractures and deltoid ligament tears.

CHAPTER 14: NEOPLASIA & ASSOCIATED GENES

APC (Genetics) - Adenomatous polyposis of the colon gene. Typically behaves as a tumor suppressor gene, although when APC is mutated, and its functions are lost, the protein can no longer function. Don't Confuse This With: DCC, HNPCC

BCR- ALB (Genetics) - A tyrosine kinase that is created by a t(9,22) which is known as the Philadelphia chromosome. This particular chromosomal mutation is common in cases of CML.

BRCA1 (Genetics) - Gene located on chromosome 17, belonging to a class of tumor suppressors that produce a protein, which normally helps to suppress cell growth. Variations of the BRCA1 are associated with an increased risk of cancer, particularly breast cancer.

BRCA2 (Genetics) - Gene located on chromosome 17, belonging to a class of tumor suppressors that produce a protein, which normally helps to suppress cell growth. Mutations in BRCA2 produce a non-functional protein that is unable to help repair damaged DNA. High prevalence of patients with Fanconi anemia are prone to leukemia; increased risk of breast cancer.

DCC (Genetics) - Deleted in Colorectal Cancer. Tumor suppressor gene located in the 18q21 region of chromosome 18. The absence of these genes is associated with the formation of colorectal cancer. The products of these genes show significant homology to neural cell adhesion molecules and other related cell surface glycoproteins. Don't Confuse This With: APC, FAP, HNPCC

HER2/NEU; CD 340 (ERBB2) (Genetics) - v-erb-b2 erythroblastic leukemia viral oncogene homolog 2; notable in its role in breast Cancer; target for breast cancer treatment. Don't Confuse This With: BRCA1, BRCA2

HNPCC (Genetics) - Hereditary Nonpolyposis Colorectal Cancer Syndrome: See Lynch's Syndrome. Don't Confuse This With: Lynch-Wiersma Syndrome

Kaposi Sarcoma (Pathology) - Vascular tumor that is the most common neoplasm in AIDS patients. Caused by Kaposi sarcoma herpesvirus or HHV-8. Lesions affect skin, mucous membranes, GI tract, lungs and lymph nodes, and contain spindle cells. Don't Confuse This With: Hemangioendothelioma, hemangioma, Henoch-Schönlein purpura

Li-Fraumeni Syndrome (Pathology) - This is an autosomal dominant disorder that results in germ line mutations of the p53 tumor suppressor gene. This means that every cell in the adult patient has this mutation and as result, the patient's susceptibility to various cancers is dramatically increased.

Mantle Cell Lymphoma (Pathology) - A non-Hodgkin's, B cell neoplasm in adults due to a t(11;14) translocation, which may be mistaken for other lymphoproliferative disorders histologically and has a poor prognosis

Non-Hodgkin Lymphoma (Pathology) - Any lymphoma that is not a Hodgkin lymphoma. Classified by tumor grade and cytological subtype. Don't Confuse This With: Hodgkin Lymphoma

Orphan Annie Eye Nuclei (Pathology) - Also known as ground-glass nuclei. These cells are a characteristic finding in a papillary carcinoma of the thyroid. The cells have very fine chromatin in their nuclei, which results in their clear appearance. Don't Confuse This With: Owl Eye Nuclei

p53 (Genetics) - Gene which encodes tumor protein p53, which responds to cellular stresses in order to regulate target genes that induce cell cycle arrest, apoptosis, DNA repair or change in metabolism. Mutants of p53 cause a loss of tumor suppressor activity, resulting in a frequent occurrence of a number of different human cancers; esophageal cancer, oral squamous cell carcinoma, hereditary adrenocortical carcinoma and lung cancer. Don't Confuse This With: TRP53; LFs1

Paget disease of breast/nipple (Pathology) - Extension of ductal carcinoma in situ (DCIS) of the breast into the nipple. Presents as a crusting exudate over the nipple and areola that may appear to be eczema. Don't Confuse This With: Paget disease of bone, Paget disease of vulva

Psammoma Body (Pathology) - These structures are located on the tips of papillae and are composed of concentrically laminated calcified concretions. They are commonly seen in papillary thyroid carcinoma, papillary renal cell carcinoma, serous papillary ovarian adenocarcinoma (cystadenocarcinoma), endometrial adenocarcinoma, meningioma, and mesothelioma.

RB1 (Genetics) - retinoblastoma gene. Located on chromosome 13; tumor suppressor gene; regulates cell division. Absence of RB1 leads to proliferation of cells in an uncontrolled manor, leading to the formation of tumors. In hereditary retinoblastoma, the RB1 gene is lost and children have multiple tumors in both eyes. Children with sporadic nonhereditary retinoblastoma have only one tumor in one eye.

Wilm's Tumor (Pathology) - AKA Nephroblastoma: malignant mixed tumor of childhood that simulates the normal development of the kidney and characteristically has a triphasic histological pattern of blastemia, stroma, and epithelium made of abortive tubules and glomeruli; associated with WAGR syndrome, Denys-Drash syndrome, and Beckwith-Wiedemann syndrome Don't Confuse This With: Neuroblastoma

WT-1 (Genetics) - WT1 gene is expressed in tissues during fetal development, consistent with its role in early nephrogenesis and development of gonads. The gene is also expressed in acute leukemias and in CD34+ hematopoietic progenitor cells. Acute nonlymphoid leukemias have the mutation of the WT1 gene in 10-15% of cases. Mutation results in Wilm's Tumor 1 - nephroblastoma.

ATM (Genetics) - Ataxia Telangiectasia Mutated. ATM gene makes a protein that is normally found in the nucleus of cells, where it helps control the rate at which cells grow and divide; also assists cells in recognizing damaged or broken DNA strands. Mutated ATM is a cause of Ataxia-telangiectasia. People with this disorder have two mutated copies of the gene; and instead of activating DNA repair, the defective ATM protein allows mutations to accumulate in other genes, which causes cells to grow and divide in an uncontrolled way. This type of cell growth leads to the formation of cancerous tumors.

BCL-2 (Genetics) - A family of proteins that regulate the integrity of mitochondrial outer membranes. In a diseased state, a t (14,18) translocation fuses this gene with IgH locus, leading to inappropriate expression of BCL 2; leading cause of CLL.

BCR (Genetics) - Breakpoint Cluster Region. Reciprocal translocation between chromosomes 22 and 9 produces the Philadelphia Chromosome, which is found in patients with Chronic Myelogenous Leukemia. The Chromosome 22 breakpoint for this translocation is located within the BCR gene.

c-myc (Genetics) - c-myc translocation; t(8:14); caused by EBV; results in Burkitt's Lymphoma. Don't Confuse This With: L-myc

FGFR2 (Genetics) - fibroblast growth factor receptor 2. Interaction with fibroblast growth factors; results in cascade of downstream signals, influences mitogenesis and differentiation. Mutations are high in breast cancer.

HTLV-1 (Microbiology) - Human T-lymphotropic Virus. Single-stranded RNA retrovirus that causes T-cell leukemia and T-cell lymphoma in adults. Polyclonal proliferation occurs through viral TAX proteins, which induces genetic instability and mutations in genes; causing tumor formation.

KSHV (Genetics) - Kaposi's sarcoma herpesvirus- G protein-coupled receptor. Proto-oncogene; activates to cause Kaposi's Sarcoma. Don't Confuse This With: CXCR2

L-myc (Genetics) - Proto-oncogene that becomes overexpressed in small cell lung carcinoma. Nuclear regulatory protein undergoes amplification, resulting in tumor growth. Don't Confuse This With: c-myc

Lindau Tumor (Pathology) - AKA hemangioblastoma.

MEN1 (Genetics) - This gene encodes menin, a tumor suppressor. Menin plays a major role in repairing DNA and regulating controlled cell death. A mutation in the MEN1 gene can cause multiple endocrine neoplasia type 1. Without this protein, cell in the endocrine glands and other tissues can divide too frequently and form tumors.

MLH1 (Genetics) - Mismatch DNA mismatch repair gene. Mutation leads to microsatellite instability. Resulting disease is HNPCC. Don't Confuse This With: FCC2; COCA2;HNPCC; MLH1

MSH2 (Genetics) - Gene provides instructions for making a protein that plays an essential role in DNA repair; fixes mistakes when DNA is copied. MSH2 was identified as a locus frequently mutated in hereditary nonpolyposis colon cancer.

MYC (Genetics) - Proto-oncogene expressed in all cells; encodes for a transcription factor that regulates expression of 15% of all genes. Mutated version leads to unregulated cell proliferation and the formation of certain types of cancer (I.e. Burkitt's Lymphoma, B-CLL) Don't Confuse This With: N-MYC, L-MYC

NF2 (Genetics) - Neurofibromin 2. NF2 gene produces a protein called merlin, also known as schwannomin; found in the nervous system. Merlin functions as a tumor suppressor protein, which prevents cells from growing and dividing too fast. Somatic Mutations in the NF2 gene involve the development of multiple noncancerous tumors called schwannomas. Inactivation of the NF2 gene is also associated with meningioma and mesothelioma. Don't Confuse This With: merlin; neurofibromin 1; SCH; Schwannomin

RAS (Genetics) - Member of a family of small G proteins that bind guanosine nucleotides GTP and GDP. When mutated by a point mutation, RAS is trapped in its activated GTP state, and the cell is thus forced into a continually proliferating state.

von Hippel-Lindau disease (Pathology) - A rare autosomal dominant genetic disease with hemiangioblastomas found in the retina, spinal cord, and cerebellum. It is further associated with renal cell carcinoma and pheochromocytoma.

ABL 1 (Genetics) - The ABL proto-oncogene has tyrosine kinase activity that promotes apoptosis of cells that suffer damage to DNA. If the ABL gene were translocated from its normal location on chromosome 9 to chromosome 22, it

begins fusion with the BCR gene. The ABL/BCR hybrid within in a cell, leads to dysregulation of apoptosis, rendering a cell likely to result in CML, ALL, T-ALL.

Bethesda classification (Pathology) - System of classification of cervical cytological smears. Separated into two categories: Low-grade intraepithelial lesion (LSIL), which corresponds to CIN I; High-grade intraepithelial lesion (HSIL), which corresponds to CIN II and CIN III. Don't Confuse This With: CIN I, II, III

Bourneville disease (Pathology) - Also known as tuberous sclerosis is an autosomal-dominant neurocutaneous syndrome. The classic triad of mental retardation, seizures, and a facial angiofibromas is used for initial diagnosis.

CYCLIN D (Genetics) - A family of three closely related proteins termed D1, D2, and D3 that are expressed in all proliferating cell types that collectively control the progression of cells through the cell cycle. D1 gene amplification is notable in mammary carcinomas.

EGF (Genetics) - Epidermal Growth Factor. Regulates cell growth, proliferation and differentiation by binding to its receptor EGFR. Mutations causes cells, especially cancer cells, to continue dividing.

EGFR (Genetics) - Epidermal Growth Factor Receptor; most commonly associated in lung cancer and glioblastoma multiforme. Amplification of EGFR results in constant activation and uncontrolled cell division.

FGFR3 (Genetics) - fibroblast growth factor receptor 3. Mutation overactivate the fibroblast growth factor receptor 3 protein, which directs bladder cells to grow and divide abnormally. Uncontrolled cell division leads to formation of a bladder tumor.

Irish nodes (Pathology) - adenopathy in the left axilla due to metastasis

JAK2 (Genetics) - Janus Kinase 2. Gene product is a protein tyrosine kinase that is involved in cytokine receptor signaling pathways; it is required for responses to gamma interferon. Somatic mutations of JAK2 are implicated in myeloid and lymphoid malignancies; predominantly atypical CML.

JAK3 (Genetics) - Janus Kinase 3. Product is a tyrosine kinase that is involved in cytokine receptor signaling pathways. A mutation in the JAK3 domain is apparent in acute megakaryoblastic leukemia cell line CMK. Tyrosine kinas is activated in numerous malignancies, including acute myeloid leukemia.

Jewett and Strong Staging (Pathology) - Staging for the invasion and development of bladder cancer

K-RAS (Genetics) - Kirsten ras oncogene homolog. Encodes a protein that is a member of the GTPase superfamily. A single amino acid substitution is responsible for activating a mutation; transforming the protein, which is, implicated in various malignancies, including lung adenocarcinoma, mucinous adenoma, ductal carcinoma of the pancreas and colorectal carcinoma. Don't Confuse This With: C-K-RAS; KRAS; Ki-Ras; NS3

Karnofsky scale (Clinical Medicine) - Developed as a clinical scale to determine a patients response to cancer treatment and its effect on their everyday living. Rates a patients physical state and prognosis post-treatment.

Langerhans Cell Histiocytosis (Pathology) - Tumor of Langerhans cells, which are immature dendritic cells found mostly in the skin. Presentation varies but usually shows multifocal cutaneous lesions, lymphadenopathy, hepatosplenomegaly, pulmonary lesions and osteolytic bone lesions. Birbeck granules are seen in the cytoplasm of such cells. Don't Confuse This With: Multiple myeloma

Lhermitte Sign (Clinical Medicine) - The patient experiences sudden electric shocks down spine when flexing the hand.

This may be caused by multiple sclerosis, vitamin B6 or B12 deficiency, a spinal lesion, or radiation myelopathy.

Lucke Virus (Pathology) - Herpes virus associated with Lucke Carcinoma.

MDM2 (Genetics) - Negative regulator of the p53 tumor suppressor genes; inhibits post transcriptional activation of p53, rendering it inactive to sense damage to DNA, thus resulting in an increased risk of sarcoma, glioma and colorectal tumors. Don't Confuse This With: MDM4, MDMX; same family of genes

N-myc (Genetics) - Activated expression of the N-Myc gene is closely related to tumor, especially human neuroblastoma. The increase of expression in neuroblastomas is the result of an increase in the amount of nuclear regulatory protein expression. Don't Confuse This With: NMYC

NF1 (Genetics) - NF1 gene makes the protein called neurofibromin. Neurofibromin acts as a tumor suppressor protein. The mutated version produces an extremely short version of the original protein, and cannot perform its normal job of inhibiting cell division. When mutations occur in both copies of the NF1 gene in Schwann cells, the resulting loss of neurofibromin allows non-cancerous tumors called neurofibromas to form. In some rare cases, inactivation of one copy of the NF1 gene in each cell increases the risk of developing juvenile myelomonocytic leukemia. Don't Confuse This With: NF2

PDGF-R (Genetics) - Platelet-Derived Growth Factor Receptor; binds PDGF-A and B to regulate cell proliferation, cellular differentiation, cell growth and development. PDGFR gene mutation commonly seen in Gastrointestinal Stromal Tumors.

Tobias' - Pancoast Syndrome (Pathology) - A malignant neoplasm; Pancoast tumor that grows in the cervical area, putting pressure on the brachial plexus, blood vessels and cervical sympathetic nerves. Characterized by severe pain in the shoulder region, atrophy of the hand and arm muscles, Horner syndrome, and compression of blood vessels with edema.

VEGFR - 2 (Genetics) - vascular endothelial growth factor receptor 2. Gene polymorphisms are associated with the risk of recurrence in Stage II and Stage III colon cancer patients. The polymorphic genes enhance angiogenesis in patients who are at an increased risk for developing tumors. Targeting VEGFR2 may be of clinical benefit for Stage II colon cancer patients.

Von Meyenburg Complex (Pathology) - A rare liver disease whereby multiple tiny hamartomas grow in the bile ducts.

Warburg Theory (Pathology) - states that cancer development is caused by damage of respiratory mechanism of cells, thus causing multiplication with increased glycolytic metabolism

Wertheim Operation (Clinical Medicine) - Excision of vagina and lymph nodes in carcinoma of uterus.

Bcl-2 like 10 (Genetics) - encodes a protein containing a caspase recruitment domain, which has the ability to induce apoptosis. A translocation of BCL10 leads to mucosa-associated lymphoid tissue (MALT) lymphoma.

BCL3 (Genetics) - Proto-oncogene; translocation into the immunoglobulin alpha-locus seen in B-cell leukemia. Product is a transcriptional coactivator that activates through its association with NF-kappa B homodimers.

BRAF (Genetics) - v-raf murine sarcoma viral oncogene homolog B1. Gene product includes a protein belonging to a family of Serine/Threonine protein kinases that regulate MAP kinase signaling pathway used for cell division and differentiation. Mutations in BRAF are associated with non-Hodgkin lymphoma, colorectal cancer, malignant melanoma, non-small cell lung cancer, and adenocarcinoma of the lung.

CCND1 (Genetics) - cyclin D1; regulator of CDK kinase; required for cell cycle G1/S transition. Interaction with the tumor suppressor protein Rb leads to mutation, amplification and overexpression of this gene.

CDK2 (Genetics) - Cyclin-dependant kinase 2. Forms a complex with cyclin E in late G1 stage, which allows for the G1/S transition. Mutations involve cancers of the brain, lung and pancreas.

CDK4 (Genetics) - cyclin-dependant kinase 4. Forms a complex with cyclin D. Responsible for the phosphorylation of retinoblastoma gene product (Rb). Mutations are associated with tumorigenesis of a variety of cancer and multiple polyadenylation; melanoma, sarcoma, and glioblastoma.

CDK6 (Genetics) - cyclin-dependant kinase 6. Controlled by the regulatory subunits of D-type cyclins. Mutations in CDK6, leads to inability to phosphorylate and regulate the activity of the tumor suppressor protein Rb.

CREB3L2 (Genetics) - Functions as a B-ZIP transcription factor. Implicated in Low-grade fibromyxois sarcoma.

CYCLIN E (Genetics) - Cyclin E binds to CDK2 in the G1 phase of the cell cycle, which is required for the transition from G1 to S phase; The complex phosphorylates p27. Overexpression of the cyclin E protein is associated with specific mutation types in the p53 gene; causing poor survival in human breast cancer.

Dabska Tumor (Pathology) - A rare, low-grade angiosarcoma that afflicts the skin of children. It has a unique histological finding of anastomosing vascular channels with intravascular papillary outpouchings that would be similar to a glomerulus. Don't Confuse This With: AV fistulas

FOX1A (Genetics) - forkhead box O1A. Selective tumor suppressor in alveolar rhabdomyosarcomas; Translocation with PAX3.

H-RAS (Genetics) - This gene belongs to the Ras oncogene family, whose products function in signal transduction pathways. Mutations in the gene cause predisposition to tumor formation, and are implicated in a variety of cancers; bladder cancer, follicular thyroid cancer, and oral squamous cell carcinoma. Don't Confuse This With: N-RAS; K-RAS; C-BAS/HAS; CTLO

HOXA11 (Genetics) - homeobox A11. This gene is involved in the regulation of uterine development. Mutations in this gene can cause radio-ulnar synostosis with amegakaryocytic thrombocytopenia; morphogenesis; irregular expression; differentiation.

Ki-RAS (Genetics) - Family of retrovirus-associated DNA sequences originally isolated from murine sarcoma viruses. The gene has been detected in human neuroblastoma and sarcoma cell lines; and seen in lung, pancreas and colon cancer. Point mutation of the GTP-binding protein causes its disruptive effects. Don't Confuse This With: H-Ras; K-Ras; N-RAS

KLF6 (Genetics) - Kruppel-like factor 6.Tumor suppressor gene involved in human prostate cancer. Deletion mutation in one KLF6 allele is deleted in 77% of prostate cancers. The wild-type KLF6 up-regulates p21 in a p53 manner and significantly reduces cell proliferation; the tumor-derived KLF6 mutants do not. Don't Confuse This With: BCD1; CPBP; COPEB

MITF (Genetics) - Microphthalmia-associated transcription factor mutations are responsible for Waardenburg syndrome, causing a failure of the transcription factor expression in the pigmented retina and other areas, resulting in the structure unable to fully differentiate. (I.e. Melanoma)

MUC1 (Genetics) - Encodes a mucin glycoprotein that is expressed in most epithelial cells. In breast adenocarcinoma.

N-RAS (Genetics) - Neuroblastoma RAS viral oncogene homolog. An oncogene encoding a membrane protein. The protein, which has intrinsic GTPase activity, is activated to a GTP- bound form by a GTPase activating protein and inactivated to a GDP-bound form by a guanine nucleotide-exchange factor. Defects in this gene are a cause of Juvenile Myelomonocytic leukemia. Don't Confuse This With: ALPS4; N-RAS, HRAS1

NOTCH 4 (Genetics) - Notch signaling can act on mammary stem cells to promote self-renewal and proliferation; resulting in normal mammary development. Notch acts as a proto-oncogene. Abnormal expression has been indicated in mammary tumors. Don't Confuse This With: MTACR1

p21 (Genetics) - Cyclin-dependant kinase inhibitor 1A; Cip/Kip family. The encoded protein binds to and inhibits the activity of cyclin- CDK2 or CDK4 complexes, and thus functions as a regulator of cell cycle progression at G1. Loss of function mutations alter the activity of p53, through which this protein mediates the p53-dependant cell cycle G1 phase arrest in response to a variety of stress stimuli. Don't Confuse This With: Cip1, CDKN1A

RBM15 (Genetics) - RNA binding motif protein 15. RBM15 is the fusion partner with MKL in the t(1;22) translocation of acute megakaryoblastic leukemia.

RET (Genetics) - ret proto-oncogene. Essential for the normal development of nerve cells; enteric neurons in the intestine and autonomic nervous system; normal kidney development. Mutations in the RET gene account for multiple endocrine neoplasia and Hirschsprung disease. Non-functional RET protein results in inability to transmits signals between cells and nerve cells to not develop properly.

Sappey, Plexus of (Anatomy) - A lymphatic network located in the areola of the nipple. Don't Confuse This With: Sappey, Veins of

VHL (Genetics) - Tumor suppressor gene that prevents cells from growing and dividing too rapidly. VHL gene makes a protein that functions as part of a complex called the VCB-CUL2 complex; which targets other proteins to degrade when the cell no longer needs them to maintain normal function. Inherited mutations cause von Hippel-Lindau syndrome. Non-inherited (somatic) mutations in this gene are associated with clear cell renal carcinoma. Noncancerous tumors such as hemangioblastomas, are also caused by the mutated gene. Don't Confuse This With: G7 Protein; pVHL; elongin binding protein

BAX (Genetics) - Gene proteins regulate apoptosis in cellular pathways involving both BCL2 and TP53. Increased BAX is associated with an increased relapse in childhood acute lymphocytic, chronic Lymphocytic Leukemia and hematopoietic malignancies.

BCL-2 like 11A (Genetics) - Normally encodes a C2H2 type zinc-finger protein, which is a common site of retroviral integration in myeloid leukemia. Translocation interaction with BCL 6 is involved in lymphoma pathogenesis.

BCL6 (Genetics) - B Cell non-Hodgkin Lymphoma (B-NHL) carry the greatest number of translocations involving the BCL6 gene locus. 15-40% of Diffuse Large B-Cell Lymphomas, 6-15% of Follicular Lymphomas and 50% of nodular lymphocyte predominant Hodgkin Lymphomas.

BCL7A (Genetics) - Three-way Translocation with Myc and IgH directly involved in Burkitt Lymphomas Cell Line. The N-terminal region of the gene product is disrupted, which relates to the high-grade B Cell non-Hodgkin Lymphoma

BCL9 (Genetics) - Associated with B-Cell acute lymphoblastic leukemia. BCL9is the target of translocation in B-Cell malignancies with abnormalities of 1q21. Overexpression leads to pathogenic significance.

BIN1 (Genetics) - Gene product is a tumor suppressor protein that suppresses the oncogene activity of Myc, inhibits the growth of tumor cell lines, and has been implicated in cell differentiation and apoptosis. BIN1 is widely lost in breast, prostate, and liver carcinoma. Don't Confuse This With: Amphiphysin

Brill-Symmer disease (Pathology) - Follicular lymphoma

BTG1 (Genetics) - B-Cell translocation gene1, anti-proliferative. The normal gene product regulates cell growth and differentiation. The mutated version is involved in a t(8;12)(q24;q22) chromosomal translocation in B-cell chronic lymphocytic leukemia.

c-SIS (Genetics) - Proto-oncogene that codes for a growth factor that is the B chain of Platelet-derived Growth Factor. Overexpression of c-SIS causes tumorigenesis. Most commonly causes Astrocytoma.

CCND2 (Genetics) - cyclin D2; regulator of CDK kinase; required for cell cycle G1/S transition. Interaction with the tumor suppressor protein Rb leads to high expression of the gene, ovarian granulosa and germ cell proliferation. Common in ovarian and testicular cancers.

CCND3 (Genetics) - cyclin D3; regulator of CDK kinase; required for cell cycle progression through G2. Interaction with the tumor suppressor protein Rb leads to unregulated cell cycle.

CDH1 (Genetics) - cadherin 1, type 1, E-Cadherin (epithelial). Encoded protein of CDH1 is a calcium dependant

189

cell-cell adhesion glycoprotein comprised of five extracellular cadherin repeats. Mutations are correlated with gastric, breast, colorectal, thyroid and ovarian cancer.

CDH11 (Genetics) - cadherin 11, type 2, OB-cadherin (osteoblast). Gene encodes a type II classical cadherin integral membrane protein that mediates calcium-dependant cell-cell adhesion. Mutant causes a lack of adhesion; in osteoblastic cell lines, it suggests a loss of bone development function and maintenance.

EP300 (Genetics) - 300 kD E1A-Binding Protein Gene. Product encodes a protein that functions as a histone acetyltransferase that regulates transcription via chromatin remodeling. Defects are a cause of Rubinstein-Taybi syndrome and epithelial cancer.

EPS15 (Genetics) - epidermal growth factor receptor pathway substrate. Its protein is involved in receptor-mediated endocytosis of EGF. Rearrangement with HRX/ALL/MLL gene occurs in acute myelogenous leukemias.

ERB-B1 (Genetics) - Protein found on the surface of cells; and to which epidermal growth factor binds. It is found at abnormally high levels on the surface of many types of cancer cells, causing the cells to divide excessively in the presence of epidermal growth factor. Commonly causes squamous cell carcinoma of the Lung. Don't Confuse This With: HER1; EGFR; epidermal growth factor receptor

ERB-B2 (Genetics) - This gene encodes a member of the epidermal growth factor receptor family of receptor tyrosine kinases. Amplification and overexpression of this gene is common in breast, ovarian and lung tumors.

ERB-B3 (Genetics) - This gene encodes a member of the epidermal growth factor receptor family of receptor tyrosine kinases. Overexpression of the gene product is associated with cancers, including prostate, bladder, and breast tumors.

ETV6 (Genetics) - ets variant gene 6 (TEL oncogene). The product of this gene contains two functional domains involved in protein-protein interactions. ETV6 has an involvement with chromosomal rearrangements associated with leukemia and congenital fibrosarcoma.

EVI1 (Genetics) - ectotropic viral integration site 1; Retroviral Proto-oncogene. Overexpression is associated with acute myelogenous leukemia, myelodysplastic syndrome and chronic myelogenous leukemia.

FSTL3 (Genetics) - follistatin-like 3 (secreted glycoprotein); role is involved in leukemogenesis.

FUS (Genetics) - fusion, derived from t(12;16) malignant liposarcoma. Mutations results in inability to bind both single-stranded and double-stranded DNA; inability to promote ATP-independent annealing of complementary single-stranded DNA to form double-stranded DNA.

GATA1 (Genetics) - GATA binding protein 1 (globin transcription factor). Normal protein plays an important role in erythroid development by regulating the switch of fetal hemoglobin to adult hemoglobin. Mutations in this gene have been associated with X-linked dyserythropoietic anemia and various cancer of the blood.

GATA2 (Genetics) - GATA binding protein 2. Family of transcription factors which are essential for normal erythropoiesis. Mutations result in various cancer of the blood.

HRPT2 (Genetics) - hyperparathyroidism 2. Gene will be expressed in primary hyperparathyroidism, and serves as a marker of Parathyroid Cancer. A single parathyroid adenoma is a resulting factor of overexpression of HRPT2.

HSPCA (Genetics) - heat shock 90kDa protein 1, alpha. Molecular Chaperone that plays a key role in signal transduction, protein folding, and protein degradation. HSPCA underexpression is related to breast cancer.

KISS 1 (Genetics) - The gene is a metastasis suppressor gene that suppresses metastases of melanomas and breast carcinomas without affecting tumorigenicity.

KIT (Genetics) - Encodes the homolog of the proto-oncogene c-KIT. Mutation in this gene are associated with gastrointestinal stromal tumors, and acute myelogenous leukemia. Don't Confuse This With: c-Kit; CD117

MKL1 (Genetics) - megakaryoblastic leukemia (translocation) 1. The protein encoded by this gene interacts with the transcription factor myocardin, a key regulator of smooth muscle differentiation. The gene is involved in a specific translocation event that creates a fusion of this gene and the RNA-binding motif protein-15 gene. This translocation has been associated with acute megakaryocytic leukemia.

MLF1 (Genetics) - myeloid leukemia factor 1. Involved in lineage commitment of primary hematopoietic progenitors by restricting erythroid formation and enhancing myeloid formation. Normally suppresses RFWD2/COP1 activity that activated p53 and induces cell cycle arrest. Non-functional MLF1 causes cell cycle to continue, despite irregularity of certain tumor growth.

p16INK4A (Genetics) - Tumor Suppressor gene. P16 plays an important role in regulating the cell cycle. Mutations in p16 increase the risk of developing a variety of cancers; notably melanoma, pancreatic adenocarcinoma; esophageal cancer and gastric cancer. Don't Confuse This With: CDKN2A

p27 (Genetics) - Chromosome 12; encodes a protein which belongs to the Cip/Kip family of cyclin dependent kinase inhibitor proteins. Major function is to stop or slow down the cell division cycle. Point mutations in p27 play a role in the development of breast cancer. Don't Confuse This With: Kip1

PBX1 (Genetics) - pre-B-cell leukemia transcription factor 1. Inactivation disrupts pancreas development; leading to unregulated pancreatic morphogenesis and differentiation.

PTEN (Genetics) - Phosphatase and tensin homolog; protein encoded by gene PTEN. It acts as a tumor suppressor through the action of its phosphatase protein product; phosphatase is involved in the regulation of the cell cycle, preventing cells from growing and dividing too rapidly. Gene is mutated in a large number of cancers at a high frequency. Inactivation of enzymatic activity is commonly found in glioblastoma, endometrial cancer, and prostate cancer.

REL (Genetics) - v-rel reticuloendotheliosis viral oncogene homolog 1. REL encodes a transcription factor that is a member of the REL/NFKB family. Normally functions to regulate genes involved in cell-cell interaction, intracellular communication, cell recruitment or transmigration, amplification of pathogenic signals, cell apoptosis and initiation of tumorigenesis. REL is implicated in cancer. Rearrangement of the rel gene results in deletion of its domain, and lymphoma formation.

RhoA (Genetics) - Ras homolog gene family; member A. Small GTPase protein that normally regulates the actin cytoskeleton in the formation of stress fibers. RhoA serves as a target for induction of vectors of certain viruses. Without a regulated signal transduction pathway, and loss of p53 function, mutations in RhoA lead to promotion of cell motility, a feature closely associated with cancer progression to malignancy.

SOCS1 (Genetics) - suppressor of cytokine signaling 1. The gene encodes a member of the STAT- induced STAT inhibitor, also known as suppressor of cytokine signaling. Mutations of the tumor suppressor gene is indicated in classical Hodgkin lymphoma and primary mediastinal B-cell lymphoma

STX (Genetics) - STX translocation from chromosome 18 to SSX1 or SSX2 on chromosome X occurs in 90% of tumors. SSX1 translocation results in biphasic tumors while SSX2 results in monophasic tumors; predominantly occurs in spindle cells, produced a spindle cell tumor.

TAL1 (Genetics) - T-Cell acute lymphocytic leukemia 1. Plays an important role in hematopoietic differentiation. Without its normal role as a positive regulator of erythroid differentiation, it is implicated in the genesis of hematopoietic malignancies.

TPMT (Genetics) - Thiopurine methyltransferase. Encodes the enzyme that metabolizes the byproduct of the thiopurine drug AZA- 6-Mercaptopurine. AZA is the standard treatment for lymphocytic leukemia; and if TPMT is mutated, then the drug can cause toxic effects in the body.

Turcot-Després-St. Pierre Syndrome (Pathology) - It is a rare autosomal recessive disorder that causes brain tumors as well as hundreds of gastrointestinal adenomatous polyposis, particularly in the colon.

Chapter 15: Nervous System

Alzheimer disease (Pathology) - Most common form of dementia characterized by long-term memory loss, confusion, and cognitive deficits; beta-amyloid plaques (made from Amyloid protein precursor APP) accumulate outside of neurons. Don't Confuse This With: Pick Disease, Friedreich ataxia

Babinski sign (Clinical Medicine) - Primitive reflex normally present in children under 1 year of age upon plantar stimulation, characterized by extension of the big toe and abduction of the other toes; considered abnormal response in anyone over the age of 1 and indicative of an upper motor neuron lesion.

Broca area (Anatomy) - Left frontal speech area, important for articulating speech. Don't Confuse This With: Wernicke Area

Brodmann Areas (Anatomy) - Neuroanatomical classification of the cortex. Includes Broca and Wernicke areas.

Brudzinski sign (Clinical Medicine) - The involuntary flexion of the legs that occurs when the head is lifted and the neck is flexed. It is an indication of meningeal inflammation or meningitis.

Cheyne-Stokes respiration (Clinical Medicine) - An abnormal pattern of breathing characterized by cyclic pattern of ventilation between apnea and tachypnea, to compensate for changing serum partial pressures of oxygen and carbon dioxide. Don't Confuse This With: Kussmaul Respirations

Down syndrome (Genetics) - Most common chromosomal disorder; mental retardation, flat facial profile with prominent epicanthal folds; ASD heart defects; increased risk of ALL, and Alzheimer's > 35YO

Edinger-Westphal nucleus (Histology) - Accessory nucleus of the oculomotor nerve, which supplies the parasympathetics to the eye; involved in the light reflex.

Erb-Duchenne palsy (Pathology) - Tearing of the upper trunk of the brachial plexus (C5, 6) possibly due to trauma during delivery leads to a characteristic "waiter's tip" stance with the arm hanging by the side in a medially rotated and pronated position. AKA Erb Palsy, Erb paralysis. Don't Confuse This With: Erb-Westphal sign

Glasgow Coma Scale (Clinical Medicine) - Scale (1-15) assessing level of consciousness and neurological impairment through visual oculomotor responses, verbal response, and motor response.

Horner Syndrome (Pathology) - A syndrome characterized by ptosis, miosis, and anhydrosis due to a lesion of the cervical sympathetic chain

Huntington disease (Pathology) - Depression, progressive dementia, choreic movements; caudate nucleus atrophy with lower levels of GABA and Ach in brain; triple repeat disorder manifesting at ages 20 to 50. The result of a tri-nucleotide repeat expansion CAG, and causes anticipation.

Locked-In Syndrome (Pathology) - Neurological condition caused by ischemic or hemorrhagic stroke due to basilar artery embolism or thrombosis. It causes quadreplegia, facial diplegia and yet patient's consciousness is preserved.

Mad Cow Disease (Pathology) - AKA Bovine Spongiform Encephalopathy: neurodegenerative prion disease of cows, fatal and can be transmitted to humans by eating infecting cows Don't Confuse This With: Creutzfeldt-Jakob Disease

Moro Reflex (Physiology) - AKA startle reflex: when the infant extends their limbs when startled; its persistence beyond 4-5 months is indicative of neurological defects.

Negri Bodies (Pathology) - Eosinophilic cytoplasmic inclusion bodies found in rabies-infected neurons.

Papez circuit (Physiology) - This is a pathway between the mammillary bodies and the subiculum that plays a role in initial memory retention and emotions.

Ranvier, Node of (Histology) - Interval between myelin sheath of nerve fiber. Don't Confuse This With: Schwann Cell

Romberg Test/Sign (Clinical Medicine) - Diagnostic method used to test for proprioception impairment. Subject stands with feet together with eyes open, then closes them. If the patient falters during a 20-30 second period of closed eyes, the test is positive and a loss of proprioception is present. Instability during eyes open is indicative of cerebellar ataxia.

Sabin Vaccine (Clinical Medicine) - This is a vaccine made from a live, attenuated polio virus. It is administered orally for the prophylaxis of poliomyelitis. Don't Confuse This With: Salk Vaccine

Salk Vaccine (Clinical Medicine) - This is a vaccine made from an inactivated polio virus. It is administered via an injection for the prophylaxis of poliomyelitis. Don't Confuse This With: Sabin Vaccine

Schwann cell (Histology) - Insulating cell of peripheral nerves. Don't Confuse This With: Node of Ranvier

Wernicke Aphasia (Pathology) - Aka Receptive Aphasia.

Bobble head syndrome (Pathology) - Rapid rhythmic bobbling of the head that is observed in children with progressive hydrocephalus.

Creutzfeldt-Jakob Disease (Pathology) - Prion disease that generally effects the cerebral cortex (layers III to IV) leading to Rapidly progressive mental deterioration and myoclonus along with dementia, loss of memory and mental acuity and occasionally visual impairment. Don't Confuse This With: Mad Cow Disease

Frey syndrome (Pathology) - Warmth and swelling of the malar region of the face upon stimulation with food. Usually occurs following trauma or infection to the parotid gland, resulting from aberrant regrowth of autonomous fibers, with crossover of sympathetic and parasympathetic pathways. Don't Confuse This With: Chvostek Sign

Friedreich ataxia (Pathology) - Inheritable, chronic disease that starts in childhood or early adolescence and involves sclerosis of the dorsal and lateral columns of the spinal cord. Symptoms include ataxia, speech impairment, irregular movement, muscle paralysis of mainly lower extremities.

Gaucher disease (Pathology) - Most common type of lysosomal storage disease due to glucocerebrosidase deficiency; accumulation of glucocerebroside causing hepatosplenomegaly, deposition in kidney, brain, bone marrow, lungs.

Klumpke palsy (Pathology) - AKA Thoracic Outlet Syndrome. Often caused by the presence of a cervical rib or a fibrous band; this syndrome is due to compression of the subclavian artery and the inferior branch of the brachial plexus (C8, T1) resulting in atrophy of the thenar, hypothenar, and interosseous muscles, as well sensory deficits on the medial aspect of the hand and forearm.

Kussmaul Respirations (Clinical Medicine) - An abnormal pattern of breathing characterized by deep, labored tachypnea, primarily associated with severe ketoacidosis - a common sequelae of type 1 diabetes mellitus. Don't Confuse This With: Kussmaul Sign, Cheyne-Stokes respiration

Lesch-Nyhan syndrome (Pathology) - A rare X-linked recessive or spontaneous genetic disease caused by hypoxanthine-guanine-phosphoribosyltransferase (HGPRT) deficiency and overproduction of uric acid; characterized by nervous system impairment, self-injuring behavior.

Miller-Fisher Syndrome (Pathology) - A severe form of polyneuroradiculitis thought to be a variant of Guillain-Barré syndrome characterized by areflexia, ataxia, as well as ophthalmoplegia.

Morvan disease (Pathology) - AKA Syringomyelia: enlarged central canal of the spinal cord damages the spinothalamic tract fibers resulting in los of pain and temperature bilaterally in the upper extremities. Don't Confuse This With: Morvan Chorea

Rett disorder (Genetics) - An X-linked pervasive developmental disorder with only females surviving and showing progressive loss of development, severe mental retardation, autism, purposeless hand movements, and deceleration of head growth causing microcephaly. Don't Confuse This With: Childhood Disintegrative Disorder

Rinne Test (Clinical Medicine) - Auditory examination with tuning fork to determine is hearing loss is sensorineural (Air conduction>Bone Conduction) or a conductive (Bone Conduction>Air Conduction).

Rolando fissure (Anatomy) - Fissure between the frontal and parietal lobes of cerebral hemispheres. AKA Central Sulcus.

Sanger Brown Syndrome (Pathology) - A disease of the nervous system that is acquired by hereditary means. It causes bilateral atrophy of the cerebellum, which results in cerebellar ataxia.

Sherrington Law (Physiology) - States that every dorsal spinal nerve root supplies a dermatome, a particular area of skin, however, with some overlap of adjacent spinal segments.

Sturge-Weber syndrome (Pathology) - It is a rare neurological and skin disorder characterized by a port wine stain birthmark, seizures, glaucoma, mental retardation. This syndrome is caused by an arteriovenous malformation around the trigeminal nerve and superficial calcifications of the cerebral cortex.

Tay-Sachs disease (Pathology) - An autosomal recessive fatal disease, also known as GM2 gangliosidosis; accumulation of gangliosides in brain and nervous tissue due to Hexosaminidase A enzyme deficiency. Patient can present with blindness, cherry-red macula, or seizures.

von Recklinghausen disease (Pathology) - Neurofibromatosis type I. Neurofibromin defect disables its ability as a negative regulator of the Ras oncogene; the clinical presentations are café-au-lait macules, neurofibromas, optic glioma, Lisch nodules, and distinct bone lesions. Don't Confuse This With: von Recklinghausen's disease of bone, neurofibromatosis type II

Wernicke center (Anatomy) - Region located at the convergence of the parietal and temporal lobes that is essential for speech understanding and formulation, but is not directly responsible for transmission of speech impulse to vocal structures. Damage results in Wernicke encephalopathy. Don't Confuse This With: Wernicke reaction

Angelman syndrome (Genetics) - A neuro-genetic disorder causing intellectual developmental delay, seizures, sleep disturbance, half flapping, and frequent smiling and laughing. This may be caused by deletion or inactivation of genes inherited maternally on chromosome 15. Involves genomic imprinting.

Charcot Triad (of Multiple Sclerosis) (Pathology) - Nystagmus, tremor, scanning speech present in Multiple Sclerosis. Compare with jaundice, fever and right upper quadrant abdominal pain that occurs in cholangitis.

Chemke Syndrome (Pathology) - A deadly syndrome that is characterized by hydrocephalus, cerebral agyria, retinal dysplasia, occasionally, occipital encephalocele, as well as other eye abnormalities.

Coxsackie encephalitis (Pathology) - Viral encephalitis seen in infants that mainly effects the gray matter of the medulla.

Dagnini reflex (Clinical Medicine) - A reflex present in conditions of hyperreflexia. Tapping on the dorsal-radial wrist causes adduction and extension of the wrist.

Erb point (Anatomy) - Point overlying the emergence of cutaneous branches of cervical plexus 2cm above the clavicle and behind the sternocleidomastoid muscle.

Falret Syndrome (Pathology) - Unknown etiology, characterized by transitional episodes of mania and episodes of depression. A period of normal psychiatric being may be present between the two states.

Fanconi-Turler syndrome (Pathology) - A congenital disorder affecting both sexes equally; characterized by cerebellar ataxia with uncoordinated eye movement, nystagmus, dysmetria and mental retardation.

Fisher plaque (Pathology) - Occurring in Alzheimer's disease, characterized by degenerative ganglion cells and breakdown products, surrounded by glial cells.

Friedreich foot (Pathology) - Seen in Friedreich ataxia; claw foot and dorsal flexion of the toes. Don't Confuse This With: Friedreich ataxia

Galant Reflex (Clinical Medicine) - Deep abdominal reflex where tapping on the anterior superior iliac spine (ASIS), elicits contraction of the abdominal muscles and lateral flexion in newborns; testing for neurological deficits.

Graefe sign (Clinical Medicine) - Failure or hesitation of the upper eyelid to follow a downward movement when the eyeball rotates downward. Often due to abnormal regeneration of the oculomotor nerve following injury.

Hallgren Syndrome (Pathology) - An autosomal recessive condition mainly characterized by spinocerebellar ataxia, retinitis pigmentosa and deafness, along with cataracts and mental disorders.

Hallpike-Dix Test (Clinical Medicine) - An important test commonly used to see if the patient's vertigo is due to certain head movements. The patient undergoes rapid positional changes from sitting erect to the supine position, hanging their head over the side of the exam table. A positive test will illicit a paroxysmal nystagmus after about 10 seconds.

Hering nerve (Anatomy) - Afferent branch of glossopharyngeal (IX) cranial nerve to the carotid sinus.

Hoffman sign (Clinical Medicine) - Tapping on the temporal region elicits grimacing due to pain; this is due to tetany.

Holmes' Degeneration (Pathology) - Degeneration of the olivary nucleus of the cerebellum leading to ataxia.

Horton Neuralgia (Pathology) - Extremely severe, brief and recurrent bouts of pain occurring unilaterally in the temporal region, eyes and neck. Don't Confuse This With: Horton's Disease (that's type I, this is type II)

Hunt Paralysis (Pathology) - Degeneration of globus pallidus. Characterized by symptoms of parkinsonism. There is no mental loss of function and no reflex changes.

Japanese B Encephalitis (Microbiology) - Epidemic encephalitis in Japan, Siberian Russia, and Asia caused by Japanese B encephalitis virus from Flavivirus genus that is transmitted by mosquitoes.

Kehrer-Adie Syndrome (Pathology) - Impaired pupillary accommodation in which one or both pupils are affected. There may also be concurrent loss of some deep tendon reflexes.

Kennedy Syndrome (Pathology) - Ipsilateral atrophy with contralateral papilledema usually due to a frontal lobe tumor or meningioma of the optic nerve. Also present: central scotoma, anosmia, headache, forceful vomiting, and psychic changes.

Kernohan Syndrome (Pathology) - A tumor of the temporal lobe causing herniation through the tentorial notch leading to the tentorium compressing the contralateral crus cerebri. Patient presents with ipsilateral hemiparesis.

Landau-Kleffner Syndrome (Pathology) - AKA Acquired Epileptic aphasia: disorder in childhood characterized by seizures (generalized and psychomotor) and aphasia; EEG displays multifocal spikes and spike and wave discharges. Don't Confuse This With: Landau Reflex

Loewenstein Occupational Therapy Cognitive Assessment (Clinical Medicine) - Cognitive tests regarding the onset and progressive evaluation of patients with traumatic brain injury.

Renshaw Cells (Histology) - Ventral horn inhibitory interneurons which receive collateral excitatory input from alpha motor nerve axons and in turn transmit inhibitory signals to the alpha motor cell bodies.

Thevenard syndrome (Pathology) - Rare, hereditary disorder affecting both sexes and occurring commonly at puberty. Characterized by degeneration of the posterior root ganglia, causing sensory defects in the lower extremities. The lack of sensation results in ulceration of the feet and destruction of the underlying bone. Later on, sensory loss may progress to the upper extremities.

Unverricht Disease (Pathology) - An autosomal recessive disorder, characterized by myoclonus and generalized seizures, in which there is degeneration of the gray matter of the brain leading to progressive neurologic and intellectual decline.

Van Allen Syndrome (Pathology) - A hereditary neuropathic amyloidosis, average onset of age 35, involving all limbs and followed by muscle weakness, muscle atrophy, and weakened or absent deep-tendon reflexes.

Weber Syndrome (Pathology) - An infarction or tumor of the midbrain tegmentum that produces paralysis of the oculomotor nerve ipsilaterally, and contralateral hemiparesis with paralysis of the extremities, face, and tongue.

Alexander Disease (Pathology) - Is one of a group of neurologic disorders, collectively referred to as leukodystrophies, which predominantly affect the central nervous system white matter. These disorders are caused by defects in the synthesis or maintenance of the myelin sheath.

Alper disease (Pathology) - An autosomal recessive disease that causes degenerative destruction of the gray matter of the brain. Manifests in early childhood and is fatal. Don't Confuse This With: MS, encephalitis

Balint Syndrome (Pathology) - A syndrome characterized by paralysis of visual fixation, optic ataxia, impairment of visual fixation, and simultaneous agnosia; usually due to damage to the superior temporal-occipital areas in both hemispheres.

Balo Disease (Pathology) - Is a variant form of multiple sclerosis with a strong correlate to viral infections in which there's concentric rings of demyelination separated by bands of preserved myelin.

Bling Sign (Clinical Medicine) - an extensor plantar response that is elicited by pricking the dorsal surface of the big toe with a pin. This sign, if positive suggests a upper motor neuron defect.

Chaddock reflex (Pathology) - Diseases to corticospinal reflex path cause extension of the great toe upon irritation of the external malleolar skin.

Charcot Disease (Pathology) - Muscular atrophy that causes increased reflexes, spastic irritability due to a disorder of the motor tracts of the lateral columns and anterior horns of the spinal cord. Don't Confuse This With: Charcot joint, Charcot angina, Charcot gait

Cincinnati Stroke Scale (Clinical Medicine) - Assess three areas: facial droop, arm drift, and speech.

Claude Syndrome (Pathology) - Damage to the midbrain causing ipsilateral oculomotor involvement and contralateral ataxia.

Coke bugs (Pathology) - An urban vernacular that describes the hallucination that a cocaine addict imagines that they have insects under their skin.

Cotunnius nerve (Anatomy) - Nasopalatine nerve.

Crocodile Tears Syndrome (Pathology) - A rare complication of Bell's palsy which is characterized by the flow of tears on the same side of the palsy during stimulation of salivation, which is most pronounced during eating.

Dawson Encephalitis (Pathology) - Progressive degenerative disease of the CNS secondary to a chronic viral infection, most often, rubeola virus. Don't Confuse This With: Viral encephalitis

Dejerine-Roussy disease (Pathology) - A syndrome that follows a stroke affecting the posterior thalamus. Symptoms include: sensory disturbances, contralateral pain, and hemiplegic hemiataxia. Don't Confuse This With: Tabes dorsalis, myalgia

Dejerine-Sottas Neuropathy (Pathology) - An autosomal dominant disease affecting peripheral nerves. The afflicted nerves show hypertrophic neuritis, characterized by hypertrophied Schwann cells with an onion-peel myelin sheath. Symptoms vary according to nerves affected. Don't Confuse This With: ALS, Guillen-Barre syndrome

Fahr triad (Pathology) - A triad characterized by neurological symptoms, lack of functional of parathyroid gland, and symmetrical calcification of the basal ganglia.

Feinberg syndrome (Pathology) - Not a term currently used. Indicates many forms of neurological atrophies, pain, and paralysis of shoulder and the cervical plexus.

Flatau-Schilder disease (Pathology) - Rare, fatal disease of the central nervous system that occurs in the late childhood;

characterized by adrenal atrophy and cerebral demyelination.

Foix syndrome I (Pathology) - A syndrome that involves the anterior portion of the red nucleus, characterized by cerebellar ataxia and hemichorea, without oculomotor nerve paralysis.

Froin symptom (Pathology) - Yellow cerebrospinal fluid that has excess lymphocytes and protein, making it prone for coagulation.

Fuchs' phenomenon (Pathology) - Upon regeneration of the oculomotor nerve (CN 3), manifestation of paradoxical lid retraction. Occurs mainly in exophthalmic goiter, but also seen after trauma, tumor compression and brainstem blood vessel damage.

Kaveggia Syndrome (Pathology) - Syndrome of unknown etiology characterized by severe mental retardation, cerebral palsy, dwarfism, and facial dystrophy.

Kleist Apraxia (Pathology) - An inability to draw, write, or build 2 or 3 dimensional objects as a result of certain types of cerebral lesions.

Krabbe disease (Genetics) - A rare, autosomal recessive degenerative disorder also known as globoid cell leukodystrophy; enzyme galactosylceramidase is deficient, causing a build up of lipid and degeneration of myelin sheath.

Kuf Disease (Pathology) - A form of sphingolipidosis that presents during adolescents. Major symptoms are mental retardation, muscle rigidity, epileptic seizures, myoclonic jerks and ataxia.

Lafora Body (Pathology) - Intracytoplasmic inclusion body consisting of acid mucopolysaccharides located intraneurally; present in familial myoclonus epileptic cases.

Meynert Cells (Histology) - Type of large pyramidal cell found in the primary visual cortex.

Reese-Blodi-Krause Syndrome (Pathology) - A condition, most often found in premature infants or individual infants of multiple births, associated with retinal and cerebral dysplasia.

Scarpa Fluid (Anatomy) - Endolymph. Don't Confuse This With: Scarpa's Fascia, Foramina, Ganglion, Membrane, Sheath, Staphyloma, Triangle

Scholz-Bielschowsky-Henneberg Disease (Pathology) - A fatal disease that is associated with the dystrophy of the white matter of the brain. It is due to the deficiency of the enzyme aryl sulfatase. The progression of the disease involves paralysis, blindness, and mental retardation.

Semon Law (Pathology) - Law stating that the abductor muscles of the vocal cords will be paralyzed before the adductor muscles, following recurrent laryngeal nerve injury.

Torsten Sjogren syndrome (Pathology) - Autosomal recessive congenital disorder affecting both sexes and manifests when the child learns to walk. It is characterized by stationary spinocerebellar ataxia, congenital cataracts, hypertension, dysarthria, mental retardation, and skeletal deformities.

Van Bogaert Encephalitis (Pathology) - A rare syndrome which causes inflammation in the white matter of the cerebrum, brain stem, cerebral cortex, thalamus, and spinal cord progressively cause by a chronic infection with measles.

Warburg Syndrome (Pathology) - A syndrome characterized by hydrocephalus, cerebral agyria, retinal dysplasia, other eye abnormalities, and infrequent occipital encephalocele due to a very fatal brain abnormality.

Weber-Fechner law (Physiology) - The intensity of a situation varies by a series of equal increments as the strength of the stimulus increases geometrically.

Weigert Stain for Myelin (Histology) - Staining using ferric chloride and hematoxylin; myelin ends up blue but yellowish if degenerated.

Weigert Stain for Neuroglia (Histology) - Similar process and stain for fibrin, whereby neuroglia and nuclei end up blue.

Austin disease (Pathology) - An autosomal recessive disease characterized by neurodegeneration in infancy. It is due to multiple sulfatase deficiency that leads to metachromatic leukodystrophy.

Avellis paralysis syndrome (Pathology) - A neurological disease resulting from occlusion of the vertebral artery in the vicinity of the brainstem. Symptoms include unilateral vocal cord and soft palate paralysis with contralateral loss of pain and temperature sensation in the trunk and arms.

Bielschowsky disease (Pathology) - Juvenile type of lipofuscinosis or cerebral sphingolipidosis.

Charcot Gait (Pathology) - A gait resulting from hereditary problems with movement control. Don't Confuse This With: Charcot joint, Charcot angina, Charcot disease

Cotard syndrome (Pathology) - Psychotic depression with suicidal impulses.

Cotte operation (Clinical Medicine) - Cutting of the presacral nerve to relieve severe dysmenorrhea.

Diallinas-Amalric Syndrome (Pathology) - A childhood disease involving nerve deafness and visual disturbances. Inheritance and etiology is unknown, but the trait is familial. Don't Confuse This With: Meniere disease

Eichorst Neuritis (Pathology) - Inflammation of the connective tissue sheath of a nerve and the interstitial muscle is affected. Don't Confuse This With: interstitial neuritis

Ekbom Syndrome (Pathology) - Neurologic disorder where there is discomfort in the legs and an urge to move them in order to relive the discomfort. Don't Confuse This With: Restless legs syndrome

Landry paralysis (Pathology) - See Guillain-Barré syndrome.

Landry Syndrome (Pathology) - aka Guillain-Barre Syndrome.

Legendre Sign (Clinical Medicine) - A sign of less resistance in lifting the closed eyelid of a patient with central facial hemiplegia, indicating the affected side.

Macewen Sign (Clinical Medicine) - Sign of hydrocephalus that is characterized by a hyperresonant sound upon percussion of the skull. Don't Confuse This With: Macewen Triangle

Machado-Joseph Disease (Genetics) - Autosomal dominant disease of trinucleotide repeat expansion, which leads to progressive spinocerebellar and extrapyramidal degeneration seen in young adults.

Marchiafava-Bignami Disease (Pathology) - Demyelination of the corpus callosum and necrosis of the temporal and frontal lobes seen in chronic alcoholism, especially wine drinkers.

Marinesco Succulent Hand (Pathology) - Condition observed in syringomyelia in which the hand is edematous and cold.

May-White Syndrome (Pathology) - a myoclonus epilepsy with accompanying deafness, ataxia, and lipomas.

Morvan Chorea (Pathology) - Fibrillary chorea; neuromyotonia with pain, severe insomnia, and excess secretions; voltage-gated K+ channel antibodies associated. Don't Confuse This With: Morvan Disease

Muller Law (Physiology) - States that each sensory nerve corresponds to a unique sensation determined by the corresponding part of the brain in which the nerve fiber terminates. Don't Confuse This With: Muller's Sign

Neuhäuser Syndrome (Pathology) - Genetic disorder characterized by mental retardation, motor disturbances (i.e.. reduced muscle tone), eye and facial abnormalities.

Nipah Virus (Microbiology) - A paramyxovirus that is the causative agent for a fatal encephalitis and meningitis. However, symptoms initially present as flu-like.

Oppenheim Reflex (Physiology) - Sign of cerebral irritation elicited by scratching the inner leg; positive if toes extend in response. Don't Confuse This With: Oppenheim Disease

Riley-Day Syndrome (Pathology) - Rare autosomal recessive disorder seen in Ashkenazi characterized by numerous autonomic (decreased lacrimation, hyporeflexia, dysphagia, inadequate blood pressure regulation) and sensory abnormalities (diminished taste, pain, temperature sensation). Synonymous with familial dysautonomia. Don't Confuse This With: Riley-Smith Syndrome

Roussey-Lévy Disease (Pathology) - Autosomal dominant condition characterized by spinocerebellar deterioration causing scoliosis, truncal and sensory ataxia and muscular atrophy of the lower limbs. Hyporeflexia is also common with the possibility of a Babinski sign. Don't Confuse This With: Friedrich's Ataxia, Charcot-Marie Tooth Disease

Scarpa Ganglion (Anatomy) - The vestibular nerve's ganglion. Don't Confuse This With: Scarpa's Fluid, Fascia, Foramina, Membrane, Sheath, Staphyloma, Triangle

Schaefer-Sorenson Syndrome (Pathology) - A triad of plagiocephaly, strabismus, and torticollis.

Scholz-Greenfield syndrome (Pathology) - see Scholz-Bielschowsky-Henneberg Disease.

Scholz' disease (Pathology) - see Scholz-Bielschowsky-Henneberg Disease.

Schultze Acroparaesthesia (Anatomy) - A disorder that is characterized by the sensation of tingling, numbness, stiffness, and pain of the upper extremity.

Schut-Haymaker Syndrome (Pathology) - an autosomal dominant syndrome that involves many symptoms: spinocerebellar ataxia, spastic paraplegia, involvement of CN IX, X, XII, and some changes in both the inferior olivary nucleus and the cerebellum.

Valentin Nerve (Anatomy) - When present, this nerve is seen connecting the pterygopalatine ganglion with cranial nerve VI.

Chapter 16: Renal

Notes: Renal physiology and pathology are amongst the highest yield topics on exams. It is highly recommended that you study this chapter especially well.

Bowman capsule (Histology) - A cup-like sac of tubular nephron that envelopes the glomerulus with the afferent and efferent arterioles extending out.

Goodpasture Syndrome (Pathology) - A rare type II hypersensitivity reaction caused by anti-glomerular basement membrane antibodies that leads to the destruction of kidneys and lungs. A smooth/linear immunofluorescence pattern is seen in studies. Don't Confuse This With: Wegener's syndrome

Kimmelstiel-Wilson Nodular Lesions (Pathology) - Microscopic nodular lesions found in diabetic nephropathy; ball-like matrix deposition in the glomerulus.

Kimmelstiel-Wilson Syndrome (Pathology) - A progressive disease of the glomerular capillaries due to diabetes mellitus. It is characterized by nodular glomerulosclerosis as well as nephrotic syndrome. This is also known as intercapillary glomerulonephritis and diabetic nephropathy.

Loop diuretics (Clinical Medicine) - Diuretics that act on the ascending loop of Henle; used to treat hypertension and edema from renal insufficiency or congestive heart failure.

Spike and dome (Pathology) - Electron microscopic and silver stain description of the granular pattern found in the basement membrane for membranous glomerulonephritis.

Tram track (Pathology) - Description of subendothelial humps observed microscopically in rapid progressive glomerulonephritis (RPGN).

Wegener Granulomatosis (Pathology) - A vasculitis that involves lung and kidney damage due to circulating c-ANCA affecting small and medium-sized blood vessels. Aka Wegener's disease. Don't Confuse This With: Goodpasture syndrome

Alport Syndrome (Pathology) - An inherited progressive form of glomerular disease that is often associated with sensorineural hearing loss and ocular abnormalities. The disorder arises from mutations in genes encoding several members of the type IV collagen that leads to defective basement membranes.

Berger disease (Pathology) - A form of glomerulonephritis also known as IgA nephropathy where there's an excessive accumulation of IgA deposition in mesangium of kidneys causing hypercellular tissue and later fibrosis. Don't Confuse This With: Buerger Disease

Crescent-moon shape or crescentric (Pathology) - Microscopic finding relating to Rapid Progressive Glomerulonephritis; proliferation of epithelial cells lining the Bowman's capsule in response to fibrin leak.

Fanconi syndrome (Pathology) - A defect in proximal tubule function leading to decreased resorption of nutrients and electrolytes. Since the resorption of bicarbonate is reduced, it results in type II renal tubular acidosis. Don't Confuse This With: Fanconi anemia

Horseshoe Kidney (Anatomy) - Inferior poles of both kidneys are fused; during development, ascending kidneys are trapped under inferior mesenteric artery; association with Turner syndrome.

Loop of Henle (Histology) - a segment of the nephron that joints the proximal tubules with the distal convoluted tubules; there is a thin descending limb and a thick ascending limb.

Maple Syrup urine disease (Pathology) - Alpha-ketoacid dehydrogenase deficiency blocks degradation of branched amino acids; severe CNS defects, mental retardation, and death.

Muddy brown casts (Pathology) - Granular casts found in urine due to acute tubular necrosis.

Staghorn Calculi (Pathology) - Composed of struvite (ammonium magnesium phosphate) that can be made by urease-positive bacteria.

Albarran Test (Clinical Medicine) - A test for renal insufficiency where drinking a large quantity of water will cause a proportionate increase in the volume of urine in normal kidneys.

Bartter syndrome (Pathology) - A rare genetic hereditary defect in the thick ascending limb of loop of Henle; characterized by hypokalemia, hypochloremic alkalosis, polyuria. Don't Confuse This With: Gitelman syndrome

Bellini, Duct of (Histology) - Straight, papillary collecting duct of kidneys; located in renal cortex and connects with distal convoluted tubules.

Bertin, renal columns of (Histology) - Medullary space between adjacent pyramids, where renal cortical tissue extends.

Gitelman syndrome (Pathology) - A rare genetic disorder with defective of Thiazide-sensitive sodium-chloride co-transporter (NCCT) in distal convoluted tubules of kidney; clinically milder than Bartter syndrome. Don't Confuse This With: Bartter syndrome

Grawitz tumor (Pathology) - Also known as Renal cell carcinoma.

Fodere Sign (Clinical Medicine) - Swelling of the lower eyelids, following a complication of kidney disease.

Hartnup disease (Pathology) - Autosomal recessive disorder with a defective neutral amino acid transporter causing malabsorption of tryptophan and neutral amino acids.

Liddle syndrome (Pathology) - An autosomal dominant syndrome caused by disregulation of ENaC, epithelial sodium channel; mimics hyperaldosteronism.

Lumpy-bumpy (Pathology) - Immunofluorescent finding of immune complex deposition in mesangial cells of the glomeruli in acute post-streptococcal glomerulonephritis.

Tamm Horsfall Protein (Pathology) - Uromodulin, a protein produced in thick ascending limb of loop of Henle in defense against UTIs; excess in urine may be due to UMOD gene defect as in medullary cystic kidney disease (MCKD).

WAGR syndrome (Pathology) - A mutation of chromosome 11 causes this childhood disorder, which leads to an increased predisposition of Wilm's tumor, Aniridia (lack of iris), Gonadoblastomas, mental retardation.

Waxy kidney (Pathology) - AKA amyloid kidney. Don't Confuse This With: Waxy cast

Winter formula (Biochemistry) - Formula in calculating metabolic acidosis; $P(CO_2) = 1.5 (HCO_3-) + 8 +/- 2$.

Balkan Nephropathy (aka. Danubian Endemic Familial Nephropathy) (Pathology) - Balkan nephropathy is a chronic tubulointerstitial disease of unknown etiology. A high frequency of urothelial atypia, occasionally culminating in tumors of the renal pelvis and urethra, is associated with this disorder.

Bright disease (Pathology) - A broad historical classification of kidney disease whereby patients were found to have protein in the urine and peripheral edema, which was categorized as acute or chronic. AKA Nephritis.

Burnett Syndrome (Pathology) - AKA milk-alkali syndrome characterized by hypercalcemia and alkalosis of the blood, which may lead to calcium deposits in soft tissues and renal failure.

Gerota capsule / fascia (Anatomy) - Renal fascia; subperitoneal fascia that envelopes the kidney and adipose tissue. Don't Confuse This With: Zuckerkandl, Fascia of

Gordon Syndrome (Pathology) - Is a rare form of pseudohypoaldosteronism seen in patients with hypertension, hyperkalemia, metabolic acidosis, normal renal function, low plasma renin activity and low aldosterone concentrations.

Malpighian Pyramid (Anatomy) - Renal (medullary) pyramid. Don't Confuse This With: Malpighian bodies, capsule, stratum

Schmidt Syndrome (Pathology) - A group of autoimmune polyendocrine syndromes, characterized by autoimmune diseases against more than one endocrine organ.

Stauffer Syndrome (Pathology) - Clinical signs and symptoms of liver dysfunction due to renal cell carcinoma, including elevation in liver function test, cholestasis and paraneoplastic syndrome.

Whitaker Test (Clinical Medicine) - Pressure-perfusion test in upper urinary tract to test for obstruction to urinary flow.

Zuckerkandl, Fascia of (Anatomy) - Describing the posterior layer of the renal fascia

Abderhalden-Kaufmann-Lignac syndrome (Pathology) - An autosomal recessive condition involving a defect in amino acid transport, resulting in deposition of cysteine crystals in various body tissues. It occurs almost exclusively in children, and results in dwarfism, rickets, and renal failure. Don't Confuse This With: Homocysteinuria, rickets, achondroplasia

Albright-Butler-Bloomberg Disease (Pathology) - An X-linked recessive disease stemming from hypophosphatemia refractory to Vitamin D therapy. Symptoms and signs include: dwarfism, rickets, missing or weak teeth, and general bone deformities. Serum phosphate and calcium are low, serum ALP is high, and urinary phosphate and calcium are also high. Don't Confuse This With: Osteomalacia, osteogenesis imperfecta

Armanni-Ebstein nephropathy (Pathology) - A histological lesion in the proximal convoluted tubules of diabetic patients characterized by glycogen vacuolization.

Ask-Upmark syndrome (Pathology) - A congenital disorder of segmental renal hypoplasia resulting in malignant nephrosclerosis. Presents in childhood.

Barakat Syndrome (Pathology) - A GATA3 gene mutation in chromosome 10 causing hypoparathyroidism, sensorineural deafness, and renal disease, including nephrotic syndrome, renal aplasia or hypoplasia, vesicoureteral reflux and chronic kidney disease.

Malpighian Capsule (Anatomy) - Fibrous membrane surrounding the spleen and hilar vessels. Don't Confuse This With: Malpighian bodies, pyramid, stratum

Selivanov Test (Clinical Medicine) - A test used to check for fructosuria.

CHAPTER 17: REPRODUCTIVE

APGAR Score (Clinical Medicine) - A means of evaluating a newborn's physical condition and responsiveness on a 10-point scale on Activity, Pulse, Grimace, Appearance, and Respiration (APGAR) taken at 1 minute post birth to assess the baby's tolerance of the birth and at 5 minutes to assess the baby's adaptation to the environment; predicts morbidity in the first 28 days.

Caesarean section (Pathology) - Extraction of a fetus through an incision in the abdominal wall.

Cowdry Type A inclusion bodies (Pathology) - Eosinophilic inclusion bodies found in herpesvirus-infected cells.

Douglas, Pouch of (Anatomy) - Fold of peritoneum between the rectum and uterus. AKA rectouterine pouch.

Graafian follicle (Histology) - A mature ovarian follicle with a full sized oocyte surrounded by the zona pellucida and a layer of follicular cells permeated by antral spaces.

Kartagener syndrome (Pathology) - Also known as immotile ciliary syndrome; autosomal recessive defect in dynein protein (motor component) of cilia; associated with infertility and situs inversus.

Leydig cell (Histology) - Cells between seminiferous tubules that produce testosterone.

Mendelian Inheritance (Genetics) - Mode of inheriting certain traits over future generations through a single gene locus.

Papanicolaou (Pap) Smear (Pathology) - Cervical carcinoma screening test

Sertoli cell (Histology) - Supportive cells in the seminiferous tubules that support spermatogenesis and establish the blood-testis barrier.

Tzanck smear (Pathology) - Cytological examination of blister fluid from herpesvirus lesion. Identification of inclusion-bearing multinucleate Tzanck cells indicates infection.

Wolffian duct (mesonephric duct) (Anatomy) - Embryological duct draining the mesonephric tubules. In males, becomes the ductus deferens. In females, becomes vestigial. Don't Confuse This With: Mullerian duct

Caesarean hysterectomy (Pathology) - Uterus removal after a Cesarean section. Don't Confuse This With: Caesarean section

Chocolate cyst (Pathology) - Endometriosis of the ovary, producing blood-filled cyst. Characterized by hyperprolactinemia.

Colles fascia (Anatomy) - Fascia covering external genitalia. Don't Confuse This With: Colles fracture, Scarpa Fascia, Camper Fascia

Cowper gland (Anatomy) - Also known as the bulbourethral gland. One of two mucus-secreting glands lying alongside the membranous urethra and secrete into the spongy urethra. Don't Confuse This With: Bartholin Glands, Skene Glands

Cri-du-chat (Biochemistry) - Congenital deletion of short arm chromosome 5; microcephaly, and mental retardation with high-pitched crying, epicanthal folds and cardiac defects

Farber disease (Pathology) - Rare, autosomal recessive, lethal disease that occurs in infancy and is characterized by disturbance of fatty acid metabolism; defect in lysosomal enzymes, resulting in accumulation of ceramide in the tissues. Manifests with failure to thrive, hoarse cry, motor and mental retardation, erythematous swellings on the skin, joints, recurrent infections, cardiac and renal failure. Associated with mutation in the N-acylsphingosine amidohydrolase (acid ceramidase) 1 gene (ASAH1). Don't Confuse This With: Farber Test

Fitz-Hugh Curtis syndrome (Pathology) - A serious complication of pelvic inflammatory disease (PID) in females, typically caused by gonorrhea or Chlamydia. This condition is due to bacterial migration from the pelvis to Glisson capsule of the liver, resulting in inflammation and adhesions or scar tissue formation on Glisson capsule. In active phase of this syndrome, acute excruciating upper right quadrant abdominal pain with pleuritic pain is present. Laparoscopy shows "violin string" adhesions. Don't Confuse This With: Fitz syndrome

Gleason Score (Clinical Medicine) - Prostatic adenocarcinoma score. Based on evaluating the two predominant patterns of glandular differentiation and summing the scores. Don't Confuse This With: Glisson Capsule, Sphincter, Triad: Glissonian Cirrhosis

Leydig Cell Tumor (Pathology) - Ovarian or testicular tumor composed of Leydig cells.

Meigs Syndrome (Pathology) - Right sided hydrothorax associated with ovarian fibromas and ascites.

Mullerian duct (Anatomy) - Paired ducts running parallel to the Wolffian ducts. In females, differentiate into the fallopian tubes, uterus and part of the vagina. AKA paramesonephric duct. Don't Confuse This With: Wolffian duct

Mullerian inhibiting factor (Physiology) - Secreted by the Sertoli cell of the testes. Prevents the differentiation of the Mullerian ducts. Promotes development of vas deferens.

Sertoli Cell Tumor (Pathology) - Tumor of Sertoli cells.

Sertoli-Leydig Cell Tumor (Pathology) - Ovarian or testicular tumor composed of Leydig cells (testosterone) and Sertoli cells (inhibin, ABP).

Signet ring cell (Clinical Medicine) - Cell type found in Krukenberg tumor of the ovary. Nucleus of the cell is displaced to the periphery by a large vacuole.

Stein-Leventhal syndrome (polycystic ovarian disease) (Pathology) - Multiple cystic ovarian follicles, producing excess androgens and estrogens. Don't Confuse This With: Polycystic kidney disease

Arias-Stella phenomenon (Pathology) - An area of increased glandular activity and secretion in the endometrium of a normal or ectopic pregnancy. The glands appear hyperchromatic or abnormal, but are not neoplastic. Don't Confuse This With: Endometrial hyperplasia, endometrial carcinoma

Blue dome cyst (Pathology) - Brown to blue cysts found in nonproliferative fibrocystic change of the breast. Usually multifocal and bilateral. Don't Confuse This With: small, round, clear blue cell

Bochdalek hernia (Pathology) - A condition that is often present during infancy in which there is a hernia through the posterior diaphragm, usually on the left.

Bowen disease (Pathology) - Carcinoma in situ of the penis. Solitary, dull-red plaque-like lesion on the shaft of the penis. Associated with HPV infection. May also occur on vulva or oral mucosa. Don't Confuse This With: Bowenoid papulosis

Bowenoid papulosis (Pathology) - Carcinoma in situ of the penis. Histologically identical to Bowen disease. Presents with multiple reddish brown papules on the glans. Associated with HPV infection. Don't Confuse This With: Bowen disease

Braxton-Hicks contractions (Physiology) - Rhythmic, painless uterine contractions that occur during the course of pregnancy.

Brenner tumor (Pathology) - Benign ovarian tumor of surface epithelial origin. Consist of abundant fibrous stroma and nests of transitional epithelium.

Chadwick sign (Clinical Medicine) - Bluish discoloration of cervix, vagina and vulva. Indicator of pregnancy.

Erythroplasia of Queyrat (Pathology) - Carcinoma in situ of the penis. Presents as an erythematous plaque on the glans penis. Associated with HPV infection.

Fabry disease (Pathology) - An X-linked recessive lysosomal storage disease caused by deficiency of alpha galactosidase A enzyme; accumulation of ceramide trihexoside in blood vessels and organs.

Goodell sign (Clinical Medicine) - Softening of the cervix and vagina. Indicator of pregnancy.

Hegar sign (Clinical Medicine) - Softening of the cervical isthmus with engorgement and bluish discoloration of the uterine cervix. Indicator of pregnancy.

Hurler syndrome (Pathology) - Mucopolysaccharoidosis type I, a lysosomal storage disease due to deficient alpha-L iduronidase; build up of heparan and dermatan sulfate occurs along with progressive deterioration, dwarfism, hepatosplenomegaly, and gargoyle-like face. Don't Confuse This With: Hunter Syndrome

Kegel exercises (Clinical Medicine) - Contraction and strengthening of perineal muscles to treat urinary incontinence.

Kobelt Tubules (Pathology) - Remnants of the Wolffian ducts in females.

Latzko Cesarean Section (Clinical Medicine) - A cesarean procedure whereby the uterus is entered by paravesical blunt dissection, avoiding the peritoneal cavity.

Leopold maneuvers (Clinical Medicine) - Techniques to determine fetal position.

Littre Glands (Histology) - Multiple mucus-secreting glands lining the urethra, facilitating smooth mechanical passage of semen during ejaculation. AKA Morgagni glands.

Lubarsch crystals (Anatomy) - Crystals in testis resembling sperm crystals

Lyon Hypothesis (Genetics) - AKA Lyonization, X-Linked Inactivation.

Nagele rule (Clinical Medicine) - Rule for determining estimated date of delivery. Determined by adding 7 days to last LMP, counting back 3 months and adding 1 year.

Niemann-Pick disease (Genetics) - A group of autosomal recessive lysosomal storage diseases leading to sphingolipidoses; includes gene mutations SMPD1, NPC1 and NPC2. Don't Confuse This With: Tay-Sachs; Sandhoff-Jatzkewitz Disease

Peyronie Disease (Pathology) - Fibrosis of the soft tissue of the penis that surrounds the corpus cavernosum. This leads to a upward curvature of the penis. The cause is unknown but is thought to be associated with trauma or injury during sexual activity. This disorder is also known as Indurato penis plastica.

Prader-Willi syndrome (Pathology) - A neuro-genetic disorder characterized by polyphagia, chronic hunger, obesity, low stature, and learning difficulties. This is a birth defect as a result of inactivation of genes inherited paternally on chromosome 15. Involves genomic imprinting.

Sandhoff-Jatzkewitz Disease (Pathology) - similar to Tay-Sachs disease, but is not as common and does not affect any one ethnic group preferentially. Unlike Tay-Sachs disease, the enzymes that are absent are hexosaminidase A and B. Don't Confuse This With: Tay-Sachs disease; Niemann-Pick disease

Schiller Test (Clinical Medicine) - Used for the carcinoma of the cervix.

Schiller-Duvall bodies (Pathology) - Structures resembling primitive glomeruli, found in yolk sac tumors of the testes.

Skene glands (Anatomy) - Mucous glands in wall of female urethra.

Walsh procedure (Clinical Medicine) - Anastomotic radical retropubic prostatectomy while sparing nerves in that area.

Asherman syndrome (Pathology) - Amenorrhea due to endometrial scarring or cervical stenosis as a result of injury or disease.

Cooper testis (Clinical Medicine) - Pain in testicles resulting from neuralgia Don't Confuse This With: Cooper hernia

Couvelaire Uterus (Pathology) - Extravasation of blood into the uterine musculature.

Hicks' sign (Clinical Medicine) - Non-labor related, uterine contractions that can last for 10-20 minutes during the third trimester of pregnancy.

Hunter ligament (Anatomy) - Round ligament of the uterus. Connects the sides of the uterus to the labia majora through the inguinal canal. Don't Confuse This With: Hunter syndrome

Hunter syndrome (Pathology) - Mucopolysaccharoidosis type II, a lysosomal storage disease due to deficient iduronate-2-sulfatase (I2S); more mild than Hurler syndrome. Don't Confuse This With: Hunter ligament; Hurler syndrome

Hutchinson teeth (Pathology) - Teeth in which the incisal edge is notched and narrower than usual. Indicative of congenital syphilis.

Keller Syndrome (Pathology) - X linked disease characterized by an imperforate anus, short stature, distinct and striking personalities, mental retardation, muscular hypotonia, macrocephaly, facial dysmorphia, seizures, occasionally sensineuronal deafness.

Klippel-Trenaunay-Weber syndrome (Pathology) - It is a rare congenital disorder which results in poorly formed blood vessels and lymph vessels leading to a variety of symptoms including a triad of port-wine stain, varicose veins, and bony and soft tissue hypertrophy of extremities.

Königstein-Lubarsch syndrome (Pathology) - A rare, systemic syndrome characterized by amyloidosis of the skin and skeletal muscle as well as macroglossia.

Laurence-Moon Syndrome (Pathology) - An autosomal recessive disorder characterized by mental retardation, retinitis pigmentosa, stunted stature, hypogonadism, and night vision problems followed by central then peripheral vision loss progressively leading to blindness. Don't Confuse This With: Biedl-Bardet Syndrome

Loeb deciduoma (Pathology) - Mass of decidual tissue in uterus caused by mechanical or hormonal stimulation in the absence of a fertilized ovum.

McRobert maneuver (Clinical Medicine) - Maneuver to reduce fetal shoulder dystocia by flexing maternal hips.

Mittelschmerz (Pathology) - abdominal pain which mimicking appendicitis, due to blood from ovulation irritating the peritoneum

Morgagni Glands (Anatomy) - AKA Glands of Littre. Don't Confuse This With: Morgagni Disease, Syndrome, Globules

Mulberry molars (Pathology) - Molar with alternative depressions and nodules on crown surface. Indicative of congenital syphilis.

Noonan Syndrome (Pathology) - An autosomal dominantly inherited disorder characterized by congenital heart disease, short stature, hypertelorism, and other features reminiscent of Turner Syndrome.

Paget disease of vulva (Pathology) - AKA Extramammary Paget disease: Intraepithelial adenocarcinoma of the vulva. Rarely associated with an underlying subepithelial or submucosal carcinoma. Don't Confuse This With: Paget disease of bone, Paget disease of breast

Retzius, Space of (Anatomy) - Space between bladder and pubic symphysis. AKA retropubic space.

Saddle-Nose Deformity (Pathology) - Nose with a depressed bridge. Seen in congenital syphilis.

Saldino Syndrome (Genetics) - This is thought to be an autosomal recessive trait that results in a lethal form of neonatal dwarfism. Death occurs shortly after birth.

Sanjad-Sakati Syndrome (Genetics) - Autosomal recessive inheritance that results in hypoparathyroidism that is associated with growth retardation and facial defects.

Sampson Cyst (Pathology) - Presents with cystic endometriosis of the ovary.

Scarpa Sheath (Anatomy) - Cremasteric fascia. Don't Confuse This With: Scarpa's Fluid, Fascia, Foramina, Ganglion, Membrane, Staphyloma, Triangle

Schauta Operation (Anatomy) - The complete removal of the uterus and the adnexa by the vaginal route.

Schimmelbusch disease (Pathology) - multiple, benign cystic growths are present in the breast.

Schinzel Syndrome I (Genetics) - Is an autosomal recessive syndrome that is associated with mental retardation, peculiar facies, absence of the corpus callosum, and polydactyl.

Schinzel Syndrome II (Genetics) - Is an autosomal dominant syndrome that is associated with ulnar ray defects, hand abnormalities, microgonadism, delayed puberty, obesity, and anal atresia.

Schubert Operation (Anatomy) - Used in patients that have a congenital absence of vagina. The operation involves the making of an artificial vagina by utilizing transplants from the rectum and the anus.

Walker chart (Clinical Medicine) - Chart of comparing fetal and placental sizes.

Alfi syndrome (Genetics) - A rare genetic mutation, monosomy 9p, that results in severe physical and mental abnormalities.

Alstrom syndrome (Genetics) - An autosomal recessive, childhood syndrome characterized by obesity, nerve deafness, retinal degeneration, diabetes mellitus, and hypogonadism. Lab findings indicate hyperuricemia and elevated triglycerides and beta-lipoprotein precursors. It is extremely rare and not life-threatening, but difficult to manage. Don't Confuse This With: Laurence-Moon-Bardet-Biedl syndrome

Amann operation (Clinical Medicine) - A surgical procedure used to create an artificial vagina in the case of congenital vaginal absence. Don't Confuse This With: episiotomy

Bartholin cyst (Pathology) - Cyst caused by obstruction of excretory duct of Bartholin gland. Don't Confuse This With: Gartner duct cyst

Batten Syndrome (Genetics) - A progressive autosomal recessive disorder in which there is muscular wasting, myotonia, cataracts, hypogonadism, and mental depreciation.

Bishop score (Clinical Medicine) - Score used to determine whether labor should be induced, based on dilation, effacement, station, cervical consistency and position.

Chiari-Frommel syndrome (Pathology) - Pathological amenorrhea and lactation following pregnancy, not caused by nursing, characterized by hyperprolactinemia and pituitary adenoma.

Del Castillo Disease (Pathology) - A male disease that causes infertility. Testes are small and lack germinal cells therefore, no sperm cells are present. Don't Confuse This With: secondary infertility

Denonvillier aponeurosis (Anatomy) - Fascia that extends from the central tendon of the perineum to the peritoneum between the prostate and rectum. AKA rectovesical septum.

Denonvillier ligament (Anatomy) - Thickening of the superior fascia of the pelvic diagram. Anchors the prostate and bladder to the pubis. AKA puboprostatic ligament.

Ferguson reflex (Clinical Medicine) - Enhancement of uterine contractions due to application of pressure on the cervix and lower uterus.

Feuerstein-Mims syndrome (Pathology) - A congenital syndrome of unknown etiology affecting many organs such as the skin, eyes, and central nervous system, characterized by the formation of nevi at birth, on the face and the scalp. Some associated features might appear as mental retardation, abnormalities in the aorta, cleft palate, ocular lesions, and rib lesions.

Gartner duct cyst (Pathology) - Congenital anomaly that presents as a cyst on the lateral wall of the vagina. Remnant of the Wolffian duct. Don't Confuse This With: Bartholin cyst

Hunner Ulcer (Pathology) - Focal lesion involving the bladder wall in chronic interstitial cystitis.

Lash Operation (Clinical Medicine) - Surgical procedure removing a wedge of internal os by suturing it into a tighter canal structure. Don't Confuse This With: Lash Casein Hydrolysate Serum Medium

Levret Forceps (Clinical Medicine) - Modified Chamberlen forceps, whereby an increased curvature accommodates for the birth canal.

Litzmann Obliquity (Anatomy) - Posterior asynclitism; fetal head position such that the biparietal diameter is oblique relative to the plane of pelvis.

Marker X Syndrome (Genetics) - AKA Fragile X Syndrome.

Martin Bell Syndrome (Genetics) - AKA Fragile X Syndrome.

Mask of Pregnancy (Pathology) - AKA melasma or chloasma: pigmentation of skin, especially the face, seen in pregnancy

Mayer-Rokitansky-Kuster-Hauser syndrome (Pathology) - Absence of vagina and uterus with primary amenorrhea due to Mullerian duct agenesis.

Meadow Syndrome (Pathology) - dilated cardiomyopathy that occurs either in the final month of pregnancy or postpartum Don't Confuse This With: Meadow Dermatitis

Menkes Syndrome (Genetics) - AKA Kinky-Hair Disease: error in copper metabolism seen shortly after birth causing short kinky hair, seizures, and progressive mental decline eventually leading to death; an X-linked disorder.

Michaelis-Gutman Body (Pathology) - Rounded cytoplasmic inclusions seen in malakoplakia, a chronic infection of the renal tract.

Nabothian cyst (Pathology) - Common cysts formed in the Nabothian glands of the uterus.

Nitabuch membrane (Anatomy) - A fibrous layer between the compact endometrium and the cytotrophoblastic shell in the placenta.

Norman-Landing Syndrome (Pathology) - A ganglioside storage disorder resulting from b-galactosidase deficiency. Don't Confuse This With: Caffey pseudo-hurler syndrome

Norton operation (Clinical Medicine) - A type of extraperitoneal cesarean section (c-section performed without penetrating the peritoneum)

Prehn sign (Clinical Medicine) - Test used to determine whether testicular injury is caused by acute epididymitis or testicular torsion.

Reifenstein Syndrome (Pathology) - Is considered to be an inherited partial androgen insensitivity syndrome.

Riley-Smith Syndrome (Pathology) - Autosomal dominant disorder characterized by macrocephaly, optic disk abnormalities, and hemangiomas that are either present at birth or develop and proliferate during childhood. Don't Confuse This With: Riley-Day Syndrome

Ritgen maneuver (Clinical Medicine) - Delivery of a child's head by applying pressure on the perineum, while controlling speed of delivery with the other hand on the head.

Sakati-Nyhan-Tisdale Syndrome (Pathology) - This is a syndrome that is observed at birth and it involves multiple defects that encompass the head, limbs, heart, ears and skin.

Schenck disease (Pathology) - See Beurmann disease.

Schimmelpenning Syndrome (Genetics) - See Schimmelpenning-Feuerstein-Mims Syndrome.

Schimmelpenning-Feuerstein-Mims Syndrome (Genetics) - A congenital condition that involves multiple systems. Most commonly it involves the skin, skeleton, eyes, and the CNS.

Schinzel acrocallosal syndrome (Genetics) - see Schinzel Syndrome I.

Sims-Huhner test (Clinical Medicine) - Test for male sterility involving sampling sperm and quality of cervical mucus post-coitus.

Solomon Syndrome (Genetics) - See Schimmelpenning-Feuerstein-Mims Syndrome.

Solomon-Fretzin-Dewald Syndrome (Genetics) - See Schimmelpenning-Feuerstein-Mims Syndrome.

Walsh, Neurovascular bundle of (Anatomy) - Structure made up of capsular arteries and veins to the prostate and cavernous nerves.

Chapter 18: Respiratory

Kohn, Pores of (Pathology) - Openings between adjacent alveoli that provide means for collateral ventilation as well as allowing the passage of fluid and bacteria.

Oat Cell Carcinoma (Pathology) - AKA Small Cell Carcinoma: extremely aggressive and early metastasizing undifferentiated tumor occurring centrally in the lungs and commonly associated with paraneoplastic syndromes of ectopic ACTH or ADH production. Treatment is generally chemotherapy and radiation as opposed to non-small cell, in which surgery is a viable option. Don't Confuse This With: Squamous Cell Carcinoma

Ranke Complex (Pathology) - Primary tuberculosis lesion in the pulmonary parenchyma of children (Ghon Primary Lesion) in conjunction with lymph node involvement. Don't Confuse This With: Ghon Complex

Farmer Lung (Pathology) - A hypersensitivity pneumonitis reaction due to inhalation of biological dusts that includes Actinomyces species and occasionally from various Aspergillus species. Also known as extrinsic allergic alveolitis. Don't Confuse This With: Loffler's Syndrome

Hare Syndrome (Pathology) - A syndrome seen in patient's with a Pancoast tumor that compresses the thoracic inlet, brachial plexus and cervical sympathetic chain. Patient will present with shoulder pain, radiating towards the axilla and down the ulnar aspect of the arm and hand.

Yellow Hepatization (Pathology) - A last stage of hepatization of the lung in pneumonia when the exudates' is purulent.

Acosta Syndrome (Pathology) - Synonym for altitude sickness or mountain syndrome. Occurs 4-6 hours after arriving at an elevation of greater than 3000m. The symptoms are: hypoxia, nausea, vomiting, headache, anorexia, insomnia, irritability, impaired vision, mental capacity, and judgment.

Brock Syndrome (Pathology) - Atelectasis of the right middle lobe of the lung. Often occurs in children with a history of asthma or atopy.

Charcot-Leyden Crystals (Pathology) - Crystals found in the sputum of bronchial asthmatics resulting from eosinophilic degranulation.

Coal Workers Pneumoconiosis (CWP) (Pathology) - Accumulation of coal dust in the lungs that causes a tissue reaction, which can develop into a more serious condition known as progressive massive fibrosis.

Hagner Syndrome (Pathology) - A syndrome commonly seen in patients with bronchogenic carcinoma characterized by finger and toe clubbing, mainly long bone periosteal new bone growth, and vasomotor disturbances.

Kveim Test (Clinical Medicine) - Used to help diagnosis patients with sarcoidosis. Extract from liver, spleen or lymph node tissue get injected intra-cutaneously and, if positive, a granuloma will develop.

Lady Windermere Syndrome (Pathology) - Mycobacterial (non-TB) pulmonary disease caused by mycobacterium avium. Patients will have a chronic cough, shortness of breath, fatigue and other less specific symptoms.

Silo Filler Disease (Pathology) - Occupational disease due to inhalation of oxides of nitrogen that leads to chemical pneumonitis and pulmonary edema.

Abraham sign (Clinical Medicine) - Upon auscultation over the acromial end of the clavicle, rales can be heard in a tuberculosis patient signifying the progression to the advanced stage of the disease. Don't Confuse This With: Pneumonia

Bat-wing edema (Pathology) - Is a radiologic finding that refers to a central, nongravitational distribution of alveolar edema. It is seen in less than 10% of cases of pulmonary edema and generally occurs with rapidly developing severe cardiac failure as seen in acute mitral insufficiency.

Curschmann Spiral (Pathology) - Spirally twisted mass of mucus occurring in the sputum bronchial asthma.

Loffler Bacillus (Microbiology) - Aka Corynebacterium diptheriae. Don't Confuse This With: Loffler Syndrome

Mixed Dust Fibrosis (Pathology) - Pulmonary reaction caused by silica dust inhalation.

Sellick maneuver (Anatomy) - Used during tracheal intubation to prevent gastric contents from spilling into the pharynx. It is elicited by applying pressure to the cricoid cartilage.

Usual Interstitial Pneumonia of Liebow (Pathology) - Fibrosis and honeycombing of the alveoli following progressive inflammation; common characteristic involving collagen-vasculature.

Weeks Bacillus (Microbiology) - AKA Haemophilus influenzae.

Aufrecht sign (Clinical Medicine) - On auscultation of the suprasternal notch, diminished breathing sounds that can be heard in a patient with tracheal stenosis.

Collier lung (Pathology) - Accumulation of carbon from inhaled smoke or coal dust in the lungs Don't Confuse This With: Collier sign

Correra line (Clinical Medicine) - The shadow of the soft tissues around inflated lungs and beneath the bones of the thorax, seen on chest radiograph.

Eaton Agent (Microbiology) - Synonym for Mycoplasma pneumoniae.

Eloesser flap (Clinical Medicine) - Surgical tract created to facilitate chronic drainage of an empyema.

Ewart sign (Clinical Medicine) - Area of dullness, bronchial breathing and bronchophony, located below angle of left scapula. Found in severe pericardial effusions.

Ghon Primary Lesion (Pathology) - See Ghon Complex.

Macleod Syndrome (Pathology) - AKA Unilateral Lobar Emphysema: one lung or lobe is hypodense due to trapped air during expiration as seen in emphysema.

Mounier-Kuhn Syndrome (Pathology) - Congenital tracheobronchiomegaly predisposing the patient to chest infection and bronchiectasis.

New York Virus (Microbiology) - Type of Hantavirus that is the causative agent for hantavirus pulmonary syndrome. The white-footed mouse of the Northeast US is consider to be the vector for the disease.

CHAPTER 19: SKIN

Athletes Foot (Pathology) – AKA Tenia Pedis: a dermatophytic infection of the feet that mostly occurs in males in warmer climates, wear closed-off footwear or walking barefoot on contaminated floors (i.e.. pools and showers). Usually characterized by erythema, scaling, hyperkeratosis and bulla formation on the feet. Don't Confuse This With: eczematous dermatitis

Butterfly rash (Pathology) - Typically occurs with SLE, more common in younger females; erythematous, macular butterfly eruption pattern on the face; characterized by scaling, erosions, and crusts.

Canker Sore (Pathology) - Painful-gray based red rimmed mucosal ulceration that most commonly found in the oral pharynx of unknown etiology.

Capillary Port Wine Stain (Pathology) - Capillary dermal malformation of blood vessels; irregular in its shape, macular, pink to purple in color; mostly commonly involves the face in distribution of the trigeminal nerve; present at birth & never disappear spontaneously. Can be seen in patients with Sturge-Weber Syndrome.

Cat Scratch Disease (Pathology) - Most often caused by *Bartonella henselae* resulting from cat contact or scratch. The disease causes a self-limited regional lymphadenopathy close to the inoculation site. There are also cases of systemic involvement but are more rare in otherwise-healthy adults.

Chediak-Higashi Syndrome (Pathology) - A rare, autosomal recessive disorder in which the patient suffers from recurrent infections, partial albinism, hepatosplenomegaly, an increased risk of lymphoreticular malignancy, and multiple neurologic abnormalities including but not limited to seizures, nystagmus and mental retardation. The defect involves the LYST gene.

Cherry Angioma (Pathology) - AKA Campbell de Morgan Spots, Senile angioma: these benign lesions are fairly common and are formed by a proliferation of dilated venules that can develop anywhere on the body but are most commonly found on the trunk. Don't Confuse This With: Spider Angioma

Fifth disease (erythema infectiosum, slapped cheek) (Pathology) - Childhood disease associated with human parvovirus B19; characterized by edematous plaques on the cheeks and erythematous macules on trunk and extremities.

Koebner phenomenon (Pathology) - Psoriatic lesions that occur at sites of cutaneous trauma.

Koplik sign (Clinical Medicine) - Clusters of bluish-white spots on the buccal mucosa, characteristic of measles and appearing on the 2nd or 3rd day of infection, prior to the typical skin eruption.

Malar Rash (Clinical Medicine) - Butterfly shaped rash seen in Systemic Lupus Erythematosus. Don't Confuse This With: Malar flush

Sister Mary Joseph Nodule (Pathology) - Metastatic carcinoma to the umbilicus from organs such as stomach, colon, ovary, pancreas, breast. It may be initial presentation of underlying malignancy. Don't Confuse This With: Spigelian Hernia

Spider Angioma (Pathology) - AKA nevus araneus, spider nevus, arterial spider, spider telangiectasia, vascular spider: a form of vascular lesion characterized by a small central elevated red dot surrounded by many smaller blood vessels.

Spider angiomas are often associated with elevated estrogen levels, such as occur in pregnancy or when the liver is diseased and unable to detoxify estrogens. Don't Confuse This With: Cherry Angioma; Spider Cell

Steven Johnson Syndrome (Pathology) - A multisystemic mucocutaneous drug-induced or idiopathic reaction characterized by tenderness and erythema, following erosion and sloughing. It is often life-threatening. AKA Lyell's syndrome.

Auspitz Sign (Clinical Medicine) - Occurrence of punctuate bleeding spots due to scraping off or picking psoriasis scales of the thin epidermis above dermal papillae

Bath-itch (Pathology) - Pruritis that occurs most often in patients with polycythemia vera after taking a bath. It's associated with mast cell degranulation that gives an elevation of histamine in the blood.

Clap, The (Pathology) - Layman's vernacular for mucocutaneous infection of the genito-urinary tract, anus, rectum, and oral pharynx which is sexually transmitted. Males usually present with whitish penile discharge and females with cervical infection and are most often asymptomatic.

Fitzpatrick skin type (phototype) (Pathology) - Classification of skin color based on the capacity to develop a tan.

Lovibond Angle (Anatomy) - Angle between proximal nail fold and nail plate; less than 180 degrees except in finger clubbing patients.

Madura foot (Pathology) - Cutaneous inoculation of an organism, commonly found in soil or plant debris, resulting in painless swelling, indurations, and sinus tract formations in the foot or hand that discharge pus and if infection is severe, may require amputation.

Meissner Corpuscle (Histology) - Sensory nerve endings found on hairless skin, which respond to fine touch and are quick adapting. Don't Confuse This With: Meissner Plexus, Pacinian corpuscles, Ruffini Corpuscles

Merkel Disc (Histology) - AKA Merkel Corpuscle, tactile cell, tactile disc: sensory nerve ending found at hair follicles which respond to stationary touch and are slow adapting. Don't Confuse This With: Meckel Diverticulum

Osler nodes (Pathology) - Tender, palpable, red, hemorrhagic and infarcted lesions on the distal finger, toes, associated with subacute bacterial endocarditis.

Pacinian corpuscles (Histology) - Mechanoreceptors in the skin that are sensitive to touch and vibration. Don't Confuse This With: Meissner Corpuscle, Ruffini Corpuscles

Spitz nevus (Pathology) - Benign, dome-shaped, hairless nevus, firm with pink, tan, brown, or black appearance; usually distributed on the head and neck; recent rapid growth is usually documented; results from hyperplasia of the epidermis and of melanocytes and dilation of capillaries.

Winterbottom sign (Clinical Medicine) - Enlargement of cervical lymph nodes due to inoculation by the human African trypanosomiasis.

Bairnsdale Ulcer (*Mycobacterium ulcerans* infection, Buruli Ulcer) (Pathology) - Occurs mostly in Tropical locations, at the site (mainly the lower extremities) of traumatic inoculation of *Mycobacterium ulcerans*. The toxin released by the microbe causes necrosis and inhibits immune response

that leads to large, deep, painless ulcerations. Don't Confuse This With: nodular vasculitis; Marjolin ulcer

Becker nevus (Pathology) - Pigmented hematoma that is characterized by pigmentation, hair growth, and slight elevation of the skin surface. Usually described as light brown in color, with sharply demarcated borders most often found on the back and shoulders. It's generally considered to be benign and occurs mostly in young-aged males.

Berloque dermatitis (Pathology) - AKA Lime dermatitis, Phytophotodermatitis: a photosensitivity reaction of the skin after contact with plant oils or cologne/perfume. The skin reacts to the photoactive oils found in these compounds and causes hyperpigmented streaks. After several days of erythema they become brown patches.

Blueberry muffin baby (Pathology) - Was characteristically seen in babies with rubella infection who displayed deep blue macular-papular lesions throughout the body. It can be further attributed with the TORCH agents of congenital infections, hematologic dyscrasias and infant malignancies such as neuroblastoma and AML.

Brill-Zinsser disease (Pathology) - Is the repeated attack of epidemic typhus years after the initial episode. In contrast to acute primary infection, Brill-Zinsser disease is generally a mild illness and caused by the Rickettsia species.

Butcher warts (Pathology) - Human Papillomavirus (most common HPV 7) infection presented clinically as cutaneous warts; most commonly in butchers, meat packers, and fish handlers

Chicago Disease (Pathology) - AKA Gilchrist Disease, North American Blastomycosis: chronic systemic mycosis infection asymptomatically involving the lungs but can spread hematogenously to the epidermis causing painless ulcers on the skin and other organs.

Clark level (Pathology) - Levels of invasion of primary malignant melanoma of the skin.

Cowden syndrome (Pathology) - Rare, autosomal dominant disorder that is characterized by multiple hamartomatous tumors; neoplasm of the germ line mutation involving the PTEN tumor suppressor gene. Screening for breast and thyroid cancer is recommended if such skin lesions are noted.

Darling disease (Pathology) - Pulmonary mycosis caused by inhalation of Histoplasma spores; hematological dissemination resulting in a chronic disease affecting the mucous membrane and the skin. It is also known as Cave Disease or Ohio Valley Disease.

Fabry-Anderson disease (Genetics) - Rare, X-linked genetic disease involving an absence of enzyme galactosyl hydrolase, leading to an abnormal metabolism of glycolipids. These glycolipids accumulate in tissues and vessels, leading to kidney and other organ dysfunctions. Mostly affecting males present with skin lesions, small red spots on the lower half of the body, corneal abnormalities, recurrent fever, and peripheral edema.

Ferguson Smith syndrome (Pathology) - Autosomal dominant condition characterized by skin neoplasm's that erupt on the normal skin in the form of acne and heal spontaneously. Mainly occurs in males and most common on the face and extremities. Also known as Smith's keratoacanthoma.

Fournier Sign (Clinical Medicine) - Congenital syphilis, resulting in oral-mucosal scars following the healing of syphilitic lesions.

Gorlins syndrome (Pathology) - AKA nevoid basal cell carcinoma syndrome: a rare, autosomal dominant condition; affects mostly the skin causing multiple basal cell carcinomas and palmer pits with variable abnormalities in other systems.

Hallopeau disease (Pathology) - A chronic skin disease, extremely prevalent in females, characterized by atrophy of the skin. Patient presents with ivory colored, shiny, flat topped papules that are surrounded by an erythematous halo.

Hashimoto Pritzker syndrome (Pathology) - A benign, self-limiting disease involving idiopathic proliferation and infiltration of tissue by Langerhans cells that fuse into giant cells and form granulomas. The nodules appear around birth or soon after and resolve within a few weeks.

Hawkins keloid (Pathology) - A colorful skin disease marked by multiple pinkish growths bordered by a purplish halo. Trauma is the usual cause. Presents from adolescents to middle age.

Hebra prurigo (Pathology) - An intensely pruritic skin disease that is both chronic and recurrent. Characterized by itchy papules of the trunk and limbs. May present in infancy.

Hutchinson rule (Pathology) - It is a rule to indicate that the eye will be affected in herpes zoster infection if there is involvement of the tip of the nose as both are innervated by the nasociliary nerve.

Leiner disease (Pathology) - Generalized seborrheic dermatitis, failure to thrive, and diarrhea in the infants; due to deficiency in complement C5.

Lund-Browder Chart (Pathology) - A burn scale to determine the intensity of burns in children.

Lyell Syndrome (Pathology) - It is also known as toxic epidermal necrolysis.

Marjolin Ulcer (Pathology) - Aggressive squamous cell carcinoma that develops in previously traumatized, inflamed, or scarred skin, appearing as a non-healing ulcerative cutaneous lesion. Don't Confuse This With: Decubitus Ulcer, Sacral Decubitii

Melanosis Riehl (melanodermitis toxica) (Pathology) - Reticular confluent pigmentation of the face, neck and extremities that may coalesce together. The dermatitis is due to a contact or photosensitivity to chemicals (cosmetics, tar derivatives).

Merkel cell carcinoma (Pathology) - A rare, malignant cutaneous tumor derived from Merkel cells. The tumor involves mostly the head and extremities and spreads to regional lymph nodes. There is a high chance of recurrence.

Milker node (Pathology) - Cutaneous infections caused by parapox viruses; presents as nodules that may erode at the site of inoculation; usually involves the hands. The human is an accidental host. Self-limiting.

Nevus of Ota (Pathology) - Dusky admixture of blue and brown hyperpigmentation of the skin and mucous membrane innervated by the first & second branches of the trigeminal nerve; mostly appears in early childhood; does not regress; very common among Asian population.

Nikolsky sign (Clinical Medicine) - It is a sign seen in pemphigus vulgaris and is observed by applying pressure in the vicinity of a bulla which causes it to spread, leading to the extension of the bulla.

Ritter disease (Pathology) - It is a staphylococcal toxin-mediated disease characterized by erythema and scalding of the skin; occurs mainly newborns and infants.

Romana sign (Clinical Medicine) - Acute American Trypanosomiasis inoculation of the conjunctiva resulting in painless edema of periocular tissue. Also known as chagoma.

Ruffini Corpuscles (Histology) - Subcutaneous sensory receptors for heat located in the fingers. Don't Confuse This With: Meissner Corpuscle, Pacinian corpuscles

Unna Seborrheic Dermatitis (Histology) - A common condition that is characterized by dermal eruptions, which are scaly and macular, that primarily affects areas of increased sebaceous gland secretions especially those on the face and scalp.

Vidal Syndrome (Pathology) - A non-inflammatory disease of the skin appearing as patches of thickened skin with lichenification, progressing to a scaly texture, on the arms, abdomen, back, buttocks, and thighs.

Wickham striae (Pathology) - White lines at lesion sites of lichen planus that are best observed with a hand-lens after application of mineral oil.

Angiokeratoma of Fordyce (Pathology) - A benign disease that involves angioamas with pebbled surface that must be differentiated from superficial spreading melanoma; comprises papules that are dark red and are multiple; involves scrotum and vulva. Don't Confuse This With: Angiokeratoma of Mibelli

Angiokeratoma of Mibelli (Pathology) - A benign disease that involves angioamas with pebbled surface that must be differentiated from superficial spreading melanoma; comprises pink to dark red papules; involves elbows, knees, & dorsa of hands. Don't Confuse This With: Angiokeratoma of Fordyce

Atrophoderma of Pasini and Pierini (Pathology) - Localized and circumscribed cutaneous sclerosis; mostly on the trunk; characterized as hyperpigmented lesions that are atrophic and cannot be felt on palpation.

B-K mole syndrome (Pathology) - Familial multiple atypical melonocytic nevi syndrome where the patient has an increased risk of developing malignant melanoma and thus the patient should be monitored carefully.

Bairnsdale ulcer (Microbiology) - Skin infection caused by *Mycobacterium ulcerans*. It appears as a painless nodule in the skin and subcutaneous tissue, usually on the lower limbs. This infectious disease is also known as a Buruli or Searl ulcer.

Bazin disease (Pathology) – AKA nodular vasculitis, erythematous induration: erythematous, tender or asymptomatic subcutaneous nodules that mostly occur on the lower extremities; associated with Mycobacterium tuberculosis immune complex vascular injury; subcutaneous blood vessel vasculitis with ischemic skin changes

Beau lines (Pathology) - These are grooved lines that run across fingernails. They may be due to a temporary stop in cell in mitosis of the nail matrix due to an infection, trauma, hypocalcemia, systemic disease or chemotherapy.

Chloracne (Pathology) - Acne due to exposure to aromatic hydrocarbons.

Civatte Bodies (Pathology) - Seen in the pathologic condition known as Lichen planus where anucleated cells are seen to have degenerated in the papillary dermis.

Cockayne-Touraine Disease (Pathology) - acral blistering and nail dystrophy, leading to scar formation that may become hypertrophic or hyperplastic; occurs in childhood; abnormality in epidermal adhesion proteins leads to blistering formations.

Darier disease (Pathology) - Disfiguring, autosomal dominant disease characterized with pruritic, scaling, & crusted papules; due to premature and abnormal keratinization and loss of epidermal adhesions. It is also known as Darier-White Disease and Keratosis follicularis.

Darier-White syndrome (Pathology) - A childhood skin disease characterized by flesh-colored, greasy, keratotic papules that can become foul-smelling over time. Transmission is autosomal dominant and the condition is worsened by sun exposure. Don't Confuse This With: Hopf's syndrome

Dariers sign (Clinical Medicine) - This is a clinical sign found in people with urticaria pigmentosa or systemic mastocytosis. Itching and formation of a wheal occur when an area on the skin is stroked. This is caused by the mast cell accumulation and degranulation with the release of histamine.

Favre-Racouchot syndrome (Pathology) - Skin disease manifesting in the middle age to those who are chronically exposed to the sun. Characterized by yellowish thickening of the skin and follicular cyst formation around the eye, on the neck, back, and behind scars, caused by degeneration of elastic tissue.

Forchheimer sign (Clinical Medicine) - Petechiae on the soft palate see in Rubella and infectious mononucleosis.

Fordyce spots (Pathology) - Asymptomatic enlargement of sebaceous glands in the mucosa and genitals, appearing as small yellow spots.

Gianotti-Crosti Syndrome (Pathology) - Discrete, nonpruritic, erythematous papules on the face, buttocks, and extension surfaces of extremities that last approximately 2-3 weeks; occurs in childhood; associated with various viral infections.

Gougerot-Blum disease (Pathology) - Pinpoint hemorrhagic lesions that are located on the lower extremities and are associated with Schamberg disease.

Haber Syndrome (Pathology) - An autosomal dominant dermatologic condition of unknown etiology characterized by rosacea-like eruptions across the face and scaly lesions on the trunk and thighs. Presents around the second decade of life.

Hailey-Hailey disease (Pathology) - Rare, chronic autosomal dominant disorder characterized by blistering of the skin due an autoimmune reaction to cell surface glycoprotein. It is also known as familial benign chronic pemphigus.

Harlequin fetus (Pathology) - It is a severe form of a congenital skin disease called ichthyosis where the child is born with a very thick stratum corneum separated by deep cracks and fissures.   The name Harlequin comes from the diamond shaped scales and facial expression (similar to the costume of Arlecchino). Due to the condition, movement is limited and infection is frequent resulting in high mortality but currently, isotretinoin has been used successfully to treat these patients.

Jacquet dermatitis (Pathology) - Also known as diaper rash. It is an irritant dermatitis occurring in children due to prolonged exposure of urine, feces, soap found on diaper.

Koenen tumor (periungal fibroma) (Pathology) - Multiple, elongated or nodular tumors producing longitudinal grooves in the nail plate; associated with tuberous sclerosis.

Lanugo hair (Pathology) - Soft fine hair that covers the fetus in the womb and sheds before birth. It is also seen in premature babies and in starvation.

Letterer-Siwe syndrome (Pathology) - It is an aggressive disease with skin and internal organ involvement caused by idiopathic proliferation of histiocytes.

Lines of Blaschko (Pathology) - Patterns of skin lesions or pigment distributions in linear form on extremities, S-shaped lines on abdomen, V-shaped on back; origin hypothesized to be genetic mosaicism and embryological processes.

Lucio Leprosy (Pathology) - An acute form of lepromatous leprosy, which can produce erythematous plaques in legs, causing ulcers and scars.

Lucio reaction (Pathology) - Irregular shaped erythematous plaques, large sloughing ulcerations on the legs; complicated by a bacterial infection that occurs in those with leprosy from Mexico / Caribbean.

Majocchi disease (Pathology) - They are pinpoint "cayenne pepper" - colored annular hemorrhages which are associated with telangiectasias; due to capillaritis; common in the lower and upper extremities.

Malpighian (Stratum) (Histology) - Name describing the combination of stratum basale, spinosum and granulosum layers of the epidermis. Don't Confuse This With: Malpighian bodies, capsule, pyramid

Martorell ulcer (Pathology) - It is associated with hypertension, causing a gangrene formation due to local obliteration of arterial arteries. It is a very painful ulcer found on the anterior lateral lower extremity.

Microabcesses of Munro (Pathology) - Psoriatic lesions that are characterized by papule formation due to aggregation of neutrophils within the stratum corneum.

Mondor disease (Pathology) - It is a rare, thrombophlebitis of subcutaneous veins from the breast to the axillary; during healing may lead to shortening of the venous cord, forming puckering of the skin.

Mongolian spots (Pathology) - Gray-blue macular lesions involving the lumbosacral region; due to dispersion of melanocytes in the dermis; may disappear in early childhood; found mostly infants of Asiatic and Native American origins.

Parkes-Weber Syndrome (Pathology) - Fast flow arteriovenous or capillary-venous malformation with soft tissue and skeletal hypertrophy. It is similar to Klippel-Trenaunay-Weber syndrome.

Pustules of Kogoj (Pathology) - It is seen in pustular psoriasis. They are epidermal pustules formed by incorporation of neutrophils into necrotic epidermis.

Recurrent aphthae of Mikulicz (Pathology) - They are recurrent, painful ulcers of unknown etiology occurring in the mouth. They are commonly called canker sores and have many other names.

Sclerema adultorum of Buschke (Pathology) - Poorly demarcated scleroderma like indurations of the skin of the upper back, neck, and proximal extremities with rapid progression and onset; some association with diabetes mellitus.

Senear-Usher syndrome (Pathology) - A variant of the blistering disorder (pemphigus) where lesions are confined to seborrheic sites such as face, forehead, presternal and interscapular regions; characterized by erythematous, crusted and erosive lesions; patients have immunoglobulin and complement deposition at the dermal-epidermal junctions.

Sneddon syndrome (Pathology) - It is a rare syndrome, characterized by mottled discoloration of the skin (livedo reticularis), cerebrovascular disease and hypertension.

Usually the rash occurs prior to a stroke. It is found in systemic lupus erythematosus.

Sweet syndrome (Pathology) - It is an uncommon, recurrent skin disease characterized by painful, plaque-like inflammatory papules, associated with fever, arthralgia, and leukocytosis. It is seen in hematological and immunological diseases including leukemia, rheumatoid arthritis and inflammatory bowel diseases.

Taenzer syndrome (Pathology) - Skin disease that is characterized by formation of red papules on the eyebrows and spreading to the remaining areas of the face; associated with falling out of hair and scarring.

Tarral-Besnier disease (Pathology) - Chronic inflammatory, exfoliate disease of the skin that is characterized by dry papules surrounding hair follicles. It can affect any sex, with onset at any age.

Touraine syndrome I (Pathology) - A condition involving the neuro-cutaneous tissues and is characterized by multiple nevus cells on the skin and the leptomeninges; frequently occurs secondary to hydrocephalus internus. Don't Confuse This With: Touraine-Christ-Siemens syndrome

Touraine-Christ-Siemens syndrome (Pathology) - Rare, congenital defect of unknown etiology that manifests at birth and is characterized by lack of development of the ectoderm and mesoderm layers, resulting in lack of sweat glands. The child presents with impairment in heat regulations and heat intolerance, in addition to dry and shiny skin. Some of the facial characteristics that are common are prominence of forehead, saddle nose deformity, deformed ears, and fine short blond hair. Don't Confuse This With: Touraine Syndrome I

Uehlinger Syndrome (Pathology) - A syndrome characterized by an uneven overgrowth of the scalp, forehead, face, and extremities, along with clubbing of the digits, and elephantitis.

Vogt-Koyanagi-Harada syndrome (Pathology) - A rare, systemic disease involving melanocyte-containing organs; characterized by vitiligo, loss of melanin in the hair, uveitis, auditory abnormalities, alopecia.

von Zumbusch (general acute pustular psoriasis) (Pathology) - initiates with an abrupt onset of burning red erythema that spreads in hours with pinpoint pustules in clusters; systemic feature are very common; can be life-threatening.

Woringer-Kolopp disease (Pageoid reticulosis) (Pathology) - It is a variant of cutaneous T cell lymphoma, characterized by localized patches and plaques of proliferating neoplastic T cells that expand intraepidermally; follows excellent prognosis.

Andogskiy syndrome (Pathology) - A disease of unknown etiology where there is chronic eczematous skin lesions followed by bilateral cataracts that form in the third decade of life. Don't Confuse This With: eczema

Brazilian Pemphigus (Pathology) - AKA Fogo Selvagem or "Wild Fire" is Endemic to South America it is a dermatological autoimmune disease consisting of bulla with serous content that can easily rupture. Patients are found to have IgG auto-antibodies against keratinocytes.

Brunsting-Perry Pemphigus (Pathology) - A rare disease that mainly involves the head and neck where blisters develop and rupture easily which leads to an erosive lesion. When blisters recur they usually present at the same site.

Cobb syndrome (Pathology) - Rare disorder that consists of cutaneous angiomas in association with arteriovenous malformations in dermatomal distribution on the trunk.

Cobbler suture (Clinical Medicine) - A suture with a needle attached at both ends.

Darier-Roussy sarcoid (Pathology) - A Boeck sarcoid-like subcutaneous lesion seen chiefly on the extremities, but can be observed on other parts of the body. Histologically, it can be identified as non-caseating granulomas. The nodules may be purplish or flesh-colored, and grow slowly without ay ulceration.

Degos' acanthoma (Pathology) - A benign epidermal tumor found in older adults that appears as a elevated, reddish plaque.

Dercum disease (adiposis dolorosa) (Pathology) - It is a rare disease caused by development of lipomas (fatty deposits) in adults who are often obese. These fatty growths are tender, localized to extremities and trunk and not well circumscribed.

Devergie disease (Pathology) - An adult skin condition showing exfoliative changes with dry papules with horny plugs infiltrating the hair follicle. Don't Confuse This With: acne

Friedreich-Erb Arnold syndrome (Pathology) - Term used to describe hypertrophy of body parts in association with different disorders. Males are more commonly involved and may progress asymptomatically.

Guttate parapsoriasis of Juliusberg (Pathology) - An eruption of salmon-like papules on the skin following a upper respiratory tract infection (group A beta-hemolytic streptococci), usually asymptomatic but may be pruritic or sensitive to touch. It may heal with scarring. The pathophysiological mechanism is unknown although it is presumed to be an immune reaction triggered by a prior infection.

Jacquet erythema (Pathology) - See Jacquet dermatitis.

Meadow Dermatitis (Pathology) - An allergic reaction occurring as a result of sun exposure after the skin has been in contact with a plant. Don't Confuse This With: Meadow's Syndrome

Meleney Ulcer (Microbiology) - Skin ulcer due to the synergistic effect of a dual infection typically with an aerobic hemolytic staphylococci and an microaerophilic nonhemolytic streptococci

Mibelli Angiokeratoma (Pathology) - Small papule caused by dilated blood vessels in the papillary dermis that may produce papillomatosis, acanthosis, or hyperkeratosis. Usually on extremities of adolescent girls. Don't Confuse This With: Mibelli Disease

Mibelli Disease (Pathology) - A rare autosomal dominant disorder seen more often in males and characterized by the formation of atrophic patches, usually on the extremities, which are surrounded by an elevated keratotic border. Don't Confuse This With: Mibelli Angiokeratoma

Miescher Elastoma (Pathology) - Circular groups of papules that have undergone hyperkeratosis and have disassociated from the skin and left a bloody depression. It is associated with the connective tissue disorder Pseudoxanthoma Elasticum. Don't Confuse This With: Miescher Granuloma

Miescher Granuloma (Pathology) - It is also known as actinic granuloma. Sun exposure causes an annular eruption on the skin due to giant cells and histiocytes phagocytosing elastic fibers within the dermis of the skin. Don't Confuse This With: Miescher Elastoma

Mucha-Habermann disease (Pathology) - A rare, idiopathic cutaneous disorder characterized by erythematous, scaly papules followed by hemorrhagic and papulonecrotic lesions.

Naegeli Syndrome (Pathology) - Syndrome characterized by hyperkeratosis, hypodontia (absence of teeth), diminished sweating and skin pigmentation.

Rosenbach Disease (Pathology) - Rare skin disease caused by Erysipelothrix rhusopathiae from contaminated meat exposure. Symptoms associated include fever, ruptured skin vesicles on the hands and feet, and inflamed mucous membranes to include the body's orifices.

Rosenbach erysipeloid (Pathology) - See Rosenbach Disease.

Sabouraud Syndrome (Genetics) - This is a congenital, autosomal dominant disease, which usually presents at birth. The characteristic findings include hairs with beadlike or fusiform enlargements that cause the hair to become brittle. This eventually leads to complete loss of hair and areas other than the scalp may be affected.

Savill Disease (Pathology) - A form of inflammatory skin disease that is characterized by erythema and scaling.

Schamberg Disease (Pathology) - A disease usually affecting the males that presents as a progressive pigmented purpuric dermatitis. The affected areas are usually the lower limbs.

Seidlmayer disease (Pathology) - See Seidlmayer purpura.

Seidlmayer Purpura (Pathology) - Purpura that occurs in infants or children after infections. It is characterized by coin-like elevated lesions.

Seidlmayer-Kokardenpurpura (Pathology) - See Seidlmayer purpura.

Sutton disease (Pathology) – AKA Recurrent aphthous stomatitis: oral aphthous ulcers involving the periadentitis mucosa – commonly referred to as "canker sores."

Reference List

Books:

Beer, M.H., Porter, R.S., & Jones, T.V. (2006). *The Merck Manual of Diagnosis and Therapy. 18th edition.* Hoboken, NJ: Wiley, John & Sons, Incorporated.

Champe, P.A., Harvey, R.A., & Ferrier, D.R. (2007). *Lippincott's Illustrated Reviews: Biochemistry. 4th edition.* Philadelphia, PA: Lippincott Williams & Wilkins.

Dorland. (2007). *Dorland's Medical Dictionary. 31st Edition.* Philadelphia, PA: Saunders Elsevier.

Fauci, A.S., Braunwald, E., Kasper, D.L., Hauser, S.L., Longo, D.L., Jameson, J.L., & Loscalzo, J. (2009). Harrison's Manual of Medicine. 17th Edition. Columbus, OH: McGraw-Hill Companies.

Goljan, E.F. (2007). Rapid Review Pathology. 2nd Edition Philadelphia, PA: Mosby Elsevier.

Moore, K.L., & Agur, A.M. (2006). Essential Clinical Anatomy. 3rd Edition. Philadelphia, PA: Lippincott Williams & Wilkins

Mosby. (2006). *Mosby's Medical Dictionary. 7th Edition.* St. Louis: Mosby Elsevier.

Ramrakha, P., & Hill, J. (2007). *Oxford Handbook of Cardiology. 1st Edition.* New York: Oxford University Press.

Stedman, T.L. (1995). *Stedman's Medical Dictionary. 26th Edition.* Philadelphia: Lippincott Williams & Wilkins.

Kumar, V., Abbas, A.K., Fausto, N., & Mitchell, R. (2007). *Robbins Basic Pathology. 8th edition.* Philadelphia, PA: Saunders Elsevier.

Venes, D. (2005). *Taber's Online Cyclopedic Medical Dictionary. 21st Edition.* Philadelphia: F.A. Davis Company.

Wolff, K., Suurmond, R., & Johnson, R.A. (2005). Fitzpatrick's Color Atlas and Synopsis of Clinical Dermatology. 5th edition. Columbus, OH: McGraw-Hill Companies.

Scientific Journals:

Lynch, HT. de la Chapelle, A. (2003 Mar 6). Hereditary Colorectal Cancer. *N Engl J Med*, 348(10): 919-32.

Hutchinson, R. (1993 February). Amyand's Hernia. *J R Soc Med*, 86(2): 104–105.

Stratakis, CA. (2003 August 21). Cushing's Syndrome. *N Engl J Med Book Review*, 349: 820 (8).

Websites:

United States National Library of Medicine. (2009, Jan 20). Genetics Home Reference. Retrieved 2009 from website: http://ghr.nlm.nih.gov/

UpToDate Online. (2009). UpToDate, Inc. Referenced from website: http://www.uptodate.com/home/index.html

Index

276

www.ingramcontent.com/pod-product-compliance
Lightning Source LLC
Chambersburg PA
CBHW071402170526
45165CB00001B/146